Girls Under the Umbrella of Autism Spectrum Disorders

Practical Solutions for Addressing Everyday Challenges

Lori Ernsperger, Ph.D., & Danielle Wendel

Foreword by Liane Holliday Willey

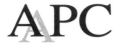

©2007 Autism Asperger Publishing Company
P.O. Box 23173
Shawnee Mission, Kansas 66283-0173
www.asperger.net

Publisher's Cataloging-in-Publication

Ernsperger, Lori.
    Girls under the umbrella of autism spectrum disorders : practical
    solutions for addressing everyday challenges / Lori Ernsperger &
    Danielle Wendel. -- 1st ed. -- Shawnee Mission, Kan. : Autism
    Asperger Pub. Co., 2007.

        p. ; cm.

        ISBN-13: 978-1-931282-47-5
        ISBN-10: 1-931282-47-1
        LCCN: 2007927796
        Includes bibliographical references and index.

        1. Autism in children. 2. Autistic children--Care. 3. Autistic
    children--Education. 4. Developmentally disabled children.
    5. Girls--Conduct of life. I. Wendel, Danielle. II. Title.

RJ506.A9 E75 2007   2007927796
618.92/85882--dc22   0706

This book is designed in Adobe Garamond and Caflisch Script.

Printed in the United States of America.

Acknowledgments

I would like to thank all of the girls with ASD and their families for sharing their unique experiences. It is my hope that we have captured your enthusiasm and knowledge to share with the world. I would also like to thank our publisher, AAPC, and Kirsten Mc-Bride for their dedication to this book on helping girls and young women on the autism spectrum.

Finally, I would like to thank my husband, Tom Ernsperger, for his continued support and encouragement through this process. And to my children, Ben and Jessica, who endured many arduous days of writing and edits. Thanks to you all for your loving support.

– Dr. Lori

A special thanks to our parents and girls with ASD who so generously shared their life experiences with us to make this book possible. Through their stories, they allowed us to enter into their worlds and walk in their shoes, if even for a brief moment.

I don't know how this book would have been possible without my friend and co-founder of our support group, Barbie Lauver. She has held my hand throughout this process by being my personal editor, confidante, and greatest cheerleader.

I would like to thank Autism Asperger Publishing Company and Kirsten McBride, our editor, for being so supportive of my first writing endeavor.

It is to my family that I owe my deepest gratitude, however. To my husband, whose inspiration enabled me to accomplish one of my dreams. To my children, who continually amazed me with their unconditional support and encouragement while I wrote this book. They allowed me to share our most intimate moments with the rest of the world.

– Danielle

Amanda LaMunyon

We would like to recognize and thank Amanda LaMunyon (11 years old with ASD) for her contributions to our book. Her amazing talent is displayed in her beautiful painting on the cover, along with her insightful story and poem. Amanda is an extremely gifted artist and has received numerous awards, such as the Temple Grandin Award and the National Volunteer Service Award. She is also a member of the Duke University Gifted and Talented Program.

In November of 2006, Amanda gave former first lady Nancy Reagan a painting of late President Ronald Reagan to be hung in his library. She also works with the Children's Miracle Network and Children's Medical Research Institute in Oklahoma and contributes a portion of her proceeds towards further research.

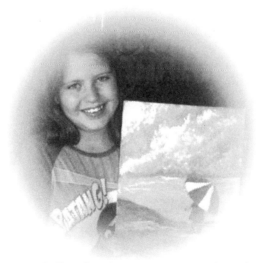

"What I like most of all is that I can encourage others through my paintings that anything is possible if you try."

– Amanda LaMunyon

Foreword

As a woman with Asperger Syndrome and as an academic in the field of pervasive developmental disorders, I can say with a good deal of authority that there is not nearly enough information on the unique ways in which autism spectrum disorders (ASDs) affect females. This is not surprising when you stop to consider that ASDs appear more obvious in males than in females – a reality that leads many to believe that girls do not represent a significant percentage of the ASD population. While it is not surprising, nonetheless, it is a dangerous supposition. Considering that the penalty females too often pay for flying under the radar is years of vulnerability and confusion that consequently leave them susceptible to additional comoribid emotional, physical, and neurological issues, one must conclude that more information on girls with ASDs is needed post haste. Thankfully, *Girls Under the Umbrella of Autism Spectrum Disorders* fills the void.

While this book does spring from the question of how ASDs present in females, it methodically goes far beyond that initial block, until an entire library of information is compiled. Just one look at the contents is proof that the book is filled with depth and scope.

The writing style is friendly, mixing creative language with timely research and applicable quotes from those intimately aware of life with ASDs. The format is user friendly. In the end, readers are provided with a comprehensive program of awareness and appropriate support models. Teachers, parents, counselors, medical professionals, and caregivers alike will benefit from reading this book, and my hunch is that everyone who reads it will turn to it again and again for additional guidance and insight.

Girls Under the Umbrella of Autism Spectrum Disorders is a terrific title because it reminds us that ASD is a wide-open reality affecting many girls with myriad possible implications, but I would like to think of the title in a different way … *Girls Under the Umbrella* paints a picture that promises a sense of protection and safety, a feeling of support and connection. This book does not let its title down.

Liane Holliday Willey, Ed.D.
Author of *Pretending to Be Normal: Living with Asperger's Syndrome* and *Asperger Syndrome in the Family: Redefining Normal*

Table of Contents

Introduction

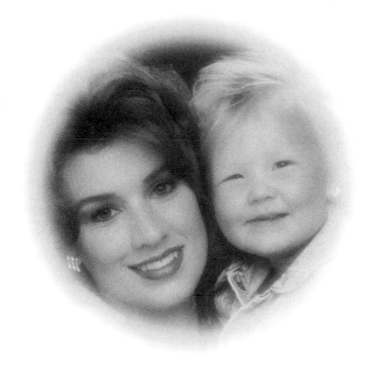

October 2000

On this mid-October afternoon, I have retreated to my backyard, a place that ordinarily would bring me peace. As I try to get comfortable in my oversized lounge chair, I look around at the empty swimming pool and leaf-covered barbecue, and I am reminded of the sounds and smell of summers gone by. I can almost hear my children giggling as they dive underwater in search of pretend buried treasures or savor the taste of a perfectly seasoned steak fresh off the grill. My heart is aching for such carefree times. How my life has changed *within just the past couple of hours. All of my dreams for my family have been altered, and I am suddenly uncertain of what the future holds.*

With my journal propped up against my legs, I can no longer hold back the tears that so desperately want to fall. I am finally able to let go after holding it together earlier today at the doctor's office for the sake of my husband and my daughter. The pages are wet from my tears, but that does not stop me from digging the pen deeper. I cannot seem to write fast enough to get the words onto the paper and out of my head.

My thoughts gradually drift to my husband. In over 10 years of marriage, we have never been at a loss for words. However, during the seemingly endless ride home from the doctor's office this afternoon, our car was eerily quiet, as if we were miles apart. The news we received weighed heavily on our minds. Upon arriving home, I was almost relieved when my husband immediately headed upstairs to be alone with his thoughts.

The neuropsychologist's office that we had just left was cold and clinical: a small room with stark white walls and uncomfortable leather chairs. As the doctor reviewed the results of our daughter's week-long testing, I began to feel the walls closing in. I couldn't focus on what she was saying. Her voice seemed so matter-of-fact when she said, "Your daughter has Asperger Syndrome." It wasn't as if the news about our daughter came as a complete shock to us. I remember spending endless hours searching for someone to tell me that there was something wrong with her. As an infant, she didn't seem to feel comfort when I held her, instead she became rigid. I felt as though she would have preferred to be left alone. She didn't respond immediately to her name being called and didn't walk until she was 18 months old. Tantrums went from zero to the boiling point in a matter of seconds, and the way she played with her toys was puzzling to me. All these concerns led to many questions. However, when we finally got them answered, I didn't want to hear.

As the doctor continued, I couldn't stop the thoughts that raced through my head. "How can our daughter be diagnosed with something we know nothing about? I don't even know how to spell it. It's not fair. How is this going to affect our family?" And then, just as quickly, I realized how very selfish I was being. "Not fair to me?" "No! It's not fair to her!" As I looked around the room I felt like my mind was in a fog, and an overwhelming feeling of loneliness and responsibility washed over me. It didn't matter that my husband was sitting right there beside me. At that time, I could only handle my own thoughts and feelings.

It felt like we had just arrived in a foreign country and had to find every road map and guidebook available to help us navigate through a place we knew nothing about. What about our daughter? We gave her this life, and now she'll have to live in it. She will need to learn the language of a place that doesn't make sense to her in order to communicate with and interpret the world as we see it. Tears came to my eyes as I thought about what kind of life she would have. What daily struggles would she have to overcome? What about the rest of our family? Will she love her brother in a way that my sisters loved me? What about our mother-daughter relationship, and all the hopes and dreams that come along with having a girl?

So began my journey with a daughter on the autism spectrum. She is more than just a "child on the spectrum;" she is a girl with Asperger Syndrome. My original questions from the day of her diagnosis have brought me down a path to a point where I am now co-writing this book about girls with autism spectrum disorders (ASD).

During the course of my research to answer all the endless questions I had, I was fortunate enough to become introduced to Dr. Lori Ernsperger. Dr. Lori is a national expert and an author on autism and other disabilities. She brings her 21 years of experience in special education and research to balance out this book. To date, almost all research in the field of pervasive developmental disorders (PDD), including ASD, has assumed that gender is irrelevant. Most researchers have taken the position that the effects of having a disability such as autism or Asperger Syndrome are the same for boys and girls, men and women, and that both groups experience the disability in the same manner, with similar experiences. Little scientific work or study has focused on the characteristics and needs of girls with ASD.

There are many compelling and wonderful stories by men and women with ASD of their personal experiences. There are also many books that report on quantitative research and best-practice strategies. In order to help both parents and professionals, we decided to combine our personal experiences with professional research to write a comprehensive book that addresses the best of both worlds.

This book was written to counteract negative stereotypes about girls with disabilities and change the field of ASD by providing girls with a voice. You will read first-hand accounts from parents, family members, and girls with ASD interspersed throughout the book. We have been very fortunate to share in the stories of some amazing and encouraging people through an ASD support group that I started in 2002. The portrayals of life experiences we have been able to capture from these families are both instructional and inspiring. The personal stories will give a glimpse of how girls with ASD understand and relate to the world and the many phases, challenges, and successes that they and their families encounter along the way. Parents, professionals, and educators of newly and previously diagnosed females from youth through adulthood will find this book very beneficial.

From the professional perspective, under the leadership of Dr. Lori, we will focus on research-based strategies and practical techniques for addressing the needs of girls on the autism spectrum. Each chapter will include descriptions of interventions and strategies developed to improve specific behaviors at home, school, and in the community.

A Brief Overview of the Book

Chapter 1 begins by defining who are girls with ASD and covers the early first signs, the diagnosis, and treatment strategies. Because parents typically are the first to recognize and question the puzzling and problematic behaviors exhibited by their children, the reader will share in the stories of other parents as they searched for answers to why their daughters interacted with and/or reacted to the world in unique ways. We will also describe why the diagnosis, although initially traumatic, often brought a feeling of relief and validation.

In addition to describing the distinct features of girls with ASD, we also suggest ways for parents and professionals to get involved in (and in some cases create) a support group. It is crucial to share our stories with others who can appreciate how overwhelming it can feel when one's child is first diagnosed with Asperger Syndrome. We will discuss my initial reactions of helplessness and fear of the life-long journey on which my family was about to embark. Like many other parents, I spent the first few months researching as many autism-related books and resources as I could and attending all conferences that I could squeeze into my already full life. I was determined that the faster and harder I worked, the quicker I could "fix" my daughter. However, upon speaking with other families in my support group, I finally came to the realization that my daughter wasn't broken; she was just different. By becoming involved in a support group, you will realize that you are not alone in this struggle.

Chapter 2 focuses on early childhood issues and behavioral concerns. We will assist parents and professionals in determining the causes of maladaptive behaviors and provide strategies for teaching replacement and alternative skills. The use of reinforcement techniques and reactive programming will also be reviewed. We will share observations and practical strategies for addressing toileting, eating, and sleeping habits.

Chapter 3 covers the school-age years (6-11 years) and reviews school placement decisions, therapy options, and social skill development for girls. The personal vignettes will reveal the difficulty in school placement and finding appropriate services. We will explore the challenging topic of sensory integration and speech and language therapy. We will also discuss the steps for preventing bullying and transitioning to middle school.

Chapter 4 targets adolescence and early adulthood (12-18 years). Here we will discuss how parents can offer information on puberty, personal hygiene, dating, and gender identity to their daughter. We will also hear from adolescent girls with ASD, who provide insight into their world as teenagers. Specific strategies will be identified for developing self-determination and self-advocacy skills. In addition, the chapter will review current trends in transitioning from high school, employment challenges, and postsecondary training. Finally, we offer advice and input from other parents and adult women with ASD with regard to the future.

Chapter 5 summarizes our findings based on extensive interviews, a review of the literature, and our personal and professional experience. We have organized the chapter around five key findings, which include promoting self-worth and independence, focusing on education, planning for the future, embracing the uniqueness of the disability, and creating a network of support in the community. It is our goal to assist parents, professionals, and girls with ASD in challenging the prevailing stereotypes of women with disabilities and assist them in navigating their journey to a successful and independent life.

Autism Spectrum Disorders, Asperger Syndrome, Pervasive Developmental Disabilities, High-Functioning Autism, Nonverbal Learning Disabilities … The List Goes On

The field of pervasive developmental disorders has grown so rapidly over the last decade that we have not had a chance to universally and irrefutably define our nomenclature. For the purpose of this book, the phrase "girls with ASD" will be generally used. We would like to define the terminology of girls with ASD as any girl between the ages of 0-21 with a diagnosis of high-functioning autism (FHA), Asperger Syndrome, or pervasive developmental disorders-not otherwise specified (PDD-NOS). Parents and professionals who work with girls with nonverbal learning disabilities (NLD) would also benefit from reading this book. Although we know there is a need for information for and about adult women with ASD, we could not adequately cover all the material for adulthood.

By Jazz (age 16 with ASD)

I want the world to know a great secret about autism spectrum disorder. This is perhaps the best kept secret in the entire world. I will tell you now, and you can tell everyone you know that you heard it here first. You got it straight from somebody who knows, right from the source:

AUTISM IS NOT CONTAGIOUS!

I have to say that, because I get strange reactions when people hear that I have autism, like it is a disease that they can catch. Some people have actually moved away from me. Others haven't called me back to babysit when they found out. I am a great babysitter, and the families who use me and know me well say that they like me because I follow the rules better than most other people. I think my autism makes me more careful. Also, my dad says that because I am creative, the kids and I get along really well. But some folks hear the word "autism" and their brains think that I am somehow dysfunctional.

CHAPTER 1

Who Are Girls with ASD?

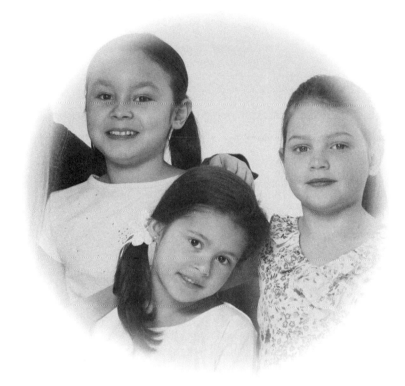

any parents of girls with ASD report spending much of the early years on an emotional roller coaster. One the one hand, they are excited and celebrate their daughter's normal developmental milestones, yet, they become increasingly concerned and anxious over puzzling behaviors.

This chapter will chronicle the stories of parents searching for answers along with their daughters' views of their unique world. We will also include the specific early first signs of ASD with the focus on girls. Finally, practical strategies will be provided for coping with the diagnosis and identifying treatment options.

First Signs

Four to one, that well-known statistic, is the reported ratio of boys to girls with ASD. Researchers have long noted that autism is more prevalent in boys than in girls – 4:1. With Asperger Syndrome, it is closer to 10:1 (Attwood, 2007; National Research Council, 2001). Although autism and Asperger Syndrome have been researched and reported on for the past 60 years, we know very little about the differences between boys and girls with these disorders.

There is an immense need to examine gender differences and the implications they may have on the diagnosis of ASD. For example, girls exhibit potential subtleties that are not detected by traditional assessment instruments and direct observations. Therefore, we need to consider whether our diagnostic criteria are too rigid or too narrow to include the symptoms of ASD in girls, which often appear "milder."

According to the American Association of University Women (AAUW, 2004), boys are only 4% more likely than girls to have a disability. Yet, they account for 68.5% of placements in special education. Boys in special education programs make up 70% of students with learning disabilities and 80% of students with emotional disturbance. The ratio of boys to girls with autism and

Asperger Syndrome placed in special education is similar. These numbers are astounding and have great implication in the education arena. The prevalence of boys in special education is evidence that the diagnostic and placement focus continues to be on the behavioral characteristics of males, often overlooking the more subtle female characteristics.

By Ashley (age 20 with ASD)

As a young child, I lived a sort of double life. To my teachers, I was a perfect, straight "A" student who was willing to help. To my parents, I was a selfish, quirky child who couldn't care less about others. Looking back, I believe I acted this way because I had a distorted view of the phrase "Treat others the way you want to be treated." I was angelic for my teachers who commended my grades, and demonic for my parents who reprimanded my unacceptable behavior. This made it hard for my parents to seek professional help for my disorder, since the rest of the world saw me as perfectly normal. At the time, Asperger Syndrome was just starting to be diagnosed in the United States. The fact that I was vicious and vile when I came home was unfathomable to everyone else who knew me. I'm not sure why I would be so cruel, but it's possible that I felt more secure and comfortable with my family and was, therefore, more likely to convey my negative feelings and actions to them as opposed to complete strangers who do not operate under unconditional love.

As this story illustrates, many young girls find a way to hide their differences and, therefore, their emotional and educational needs may not be met (Attwood, 2007). Typically developing children display gender differences at an early age. By age 6, girls have gender identified and know the differences between boys and girls (Gurian, 2002). Male-versus-female characteristics become more prevalent between the ages of 5 to 7. Researchers have suggested that because boys exhibit a higher level of activity and behavioral problems, they are more likely to be referred for special services (Rousso & Wehmeyer, 2001). It is also suggested that these differences have an impact on the overall identification and placement of girls on the autism spectrum and on them receiving special education services (Attwood, 2007).

By Jana (age 27 with ASD)

There are two types of waiting rooms: One is the Pottery Barn-esque with all the creature comforts one might expect from a shrink that charges $300 per hour, with bottled mineral water and biscottis at one's fingertips and sound makers to drown out session noise. The other is a southwestern hodgepodge disaster with threadbare armchairs, decade-old Parenthood *magazines, and harsh overhead lighting.*

During the fall of 2002, I found myself waiting and fidgeting in a hodgepodge disaster, audibly cursing my cheap medical policy. After waiting an eternity, the previous patient slipped out of the building and back into the world. Subsequent to pronouncing my name incorrectly, the doctor ushered me into the office, and I hesitantly plunked down on the beige couch, squirming to avoid the "warm" cushion. The room smelled of fear, tears, and almost-stifled gas. The doctor readied his trusty pen and asked why I was there. I was too busy judging the ve-

neer of my dingy cell, noticing that he'd graduated from some no-name university, to give the session a chance, but once we made eye contact, I crumbled.

I immediately began sobbing and relating my dismal mental health history, which at that point spanned a decade and included private sessions, hospitalizations, and residential treatment. He listened intently for 30 minutes as I ran down my laundry list of mental ailments and failed treatment. While I reached for a tissue, he seized the opportunity and speedily suggested I'd been misdiagnosed and might want to investigate Asperger Syndrome and autism. I fumbled for my checkbook, paid the man, and sped to the nearest bookstore.

The selection of books on Asperger Syndrome/autism was extremely limited at the time, but I managed to find three and read them from cover to cover within one and a half hours. Those words encapsulated my childhood, from the lack of emotional connections to social anxiety to confusion and severe depression. I'd finally found the answer to so many questions. I was at once elated and deeply saddened. My family had spent years and a fortune seeking help for me. I asked myself why none of the other doctors (with their Ivy League educations, published articles, and countless patients) ever solved my riddle. I felt sorry for myself during the next months and couldn't let go of my troubled past. In my mind, I had suffered needlessly for years and placed my loved ones in innumerably horrible situations. Despite my age and responsibilities, I wanted a second chance. To quit work and focus on myself for a couple years seemed to me the perfect answer.

Why did it take so long for Jana to receive assistance and a diagnosis? According Hans Asperger's original research (Frith, 1991), "girls are the better learners. They are more gifted for the concrete and practical and for tidy methodical work. In the autistic individual the male pattern is exaggerated to the extreme" (p. 85). Asperger goes on to say, "It may be that there are no autistic girls among our cases or it could be that autistic traits in the female only become evident after puberty. We just don't know" (p. 85).

In 1944, Asperger was questioning whether girls with ASD existed and, if so, what types of characteristics they displayed. We know that ASD is a developmental disorder, which means that characteristics and symptoms can change or vary over time. Hans Asperger may have been correct in his presumption. Some researchers have suggested that girls on the autism spectrum are diagnosed later than their male counterparts (Attwood, 2007). The specific male characteristics that Dr. Asperger was looking for were not present in the earlier years. Some of them may not be as prevalent until the school age years or adolescence. In this next story, Ashley details her adolescence with ASD.

By Ashley (age 20 with ASD)

During the adolescent stage in my life, many of my Asperger tendencies became noticeable to me, both the good and the bad. I excelled in mathematics, and had an unusually natural ability to play the flute. When I complained to my teachers about the other students pestering me, they told me that my overreactions entertained my classmates. The students could see how much their actions bothered me, so they continued to tease. My opinion was that it was rude to annoy others, regardless of their actions or the entertainment that it provided. I found it incomprehensible that my classmates could think otherwise. Because of these teachers, I am now one of the most laid-back and impossible-to-offend people on earth. I have learned to let the little things go, not let them get to me, and I have terminated the free entertainment to my peers.

There are other theories about the increased in prevalence of males with ASD. According to Jean Kearns Miller, editor of *Women from Another Planet* (2003), clinicians utilize a male-centered profile when diagnosing ASD. Therefore, when boys demonstrate aggressive, noisy, or acting-out behavior, they are more likely to be identified with a disability, whereas girls who are well behaved, compliant, and quiet may be overlooked and under-diagnosed (Attwood, 1999). Kopp and Gillberg (1992) agree that the under-diagnosing of girls with ASD is due to our reliance on the male prototype of autism, whereby diagnosis is based on behaviors that are more extreme in how they present themselves to the clinician or educator. Thus, if we examine girls who exhibit male types of externalized behaviors, they are often identified at a much earlier age than most other girls (Kopp & Gillberg, 1992). Most clinicians and educators utilize a one-size-fits-all model for diagnosis, which ignores the fact that assessment tools may not detect the characteristics or subtleties of girls with ASD.

Personality Traits and Gender Difference

We will now take a closer look at the personality traits and gender differences in boys versus girls on the autism spectrum. The well-known nursery rhyme "girls are made of sugar and spice and everything nice" can be a double-edged sword when it comes to evaluating and diagnosing girls on the autism spectrum. As Ashley explained earlier, she was a perfect student in school, and consequently the characteristics of ASD were overlooked.

In our society, girls are traditionally raised to be nice, kind, and nurturing. Historically, it has been acceptable for girls to be passive and dependent. According to Zosia Zaks' book *Life and Love: Positive Strategies for Autistic Adults* (2006), a woman on the autism spectrum, "whenever a girl acts in a sensitive manner toward the people around her and her community, she is praised and her behavior is reinforced … I discovered early that I could win people over and that they would assume I was a good girl with no problems – if I did nice things" (p. 297).

Girls with ASD tend to be more social than their male counterparts. Gillberg (in Frith, 1991) noted "ASD can occur in girls. It is suggested that on the surface the symptoms of impairment of social interaction might be less conspicuous than corresponding symptoms in boys" (p. 129). Girls have more advanced social skills, which can cover the underlying characteristics of ASD. For example, "Little girls are usually instructed and expected to talk in a pleasant manner, so girls on the spectrum may be more sensitive to criticism regarding voice and conversation skills than boys. For this reason, a boy may be more likely to jump into a conversation, not sensing he is interrupting, too loud, or missing the point. Conversely, realizing a deficit in this area, a girl may decide the best tactic is to be quiet rather than causing a scene. As a result, her conversational issues may go undetected. A girl may also be more likely to act like she "gets it" to avoid the conflict, ridicule, or danger"

(Zaks, 2006, p. 295). Our society may tolerate some of the same autistic traits in girls over boys. Kopp and Gillberg (1992) studied six girls with high-functioning ASD who had IQs from 60-100 and spoke in complete sentences. They found that the girls tended to differ greatly from their male counterparts. The symptoms appeared milder or borderline with an increase in co-morbidity with obsessive compulsive disorder, anxiety, and other schizoid symptoms.

By Karen (Mother of Rosemarie, age 17)

From the beginning, I knew that my little girl was way different from her two brothers. She was emotional, spirited, and eccentric. Her feet would twirl, her hands would shake. As we look back, my husband and I believe what we were seeing was the beginning of hand flapping and rocking. She was so difficult in every way possible. However, I knew from raising my boys that my parenting skills could not be that bad. I looked forward to my sons' first steps, first words, first everything. In comparison, Rosemarie hated to walk and would cry in order to be carried. Although she could speak, she didn't know how to use her words to communicate her needs, and would often echo back what she was hearing. We had to constantly guess what she wanted from us. She screamed when we had to go out. She screamed when we had to leave and come home. When we couldn't figure her out, which was most of the time, Rosemarie would scream sometimes for hours. I remember the many times my husband and I sat on the bed, holding this strange, screaming child, trying to keep her from throwing herself all over the place. Rosemarie was happiest when she was on the floor, wearing as few clothes as she could get away with, hovering over a huge sheet of drawing paper. Drawing became her way to communicate and escape from a world that was too complex for us to understand.

This mother's story demonstrates that some girls with ASD experience the early signs of ASD, including anxiety and communication impairment. Kopp and Gillberg (1992) found that girls demonstrated excessive worrying as they got older and more anxious. Also, the girls in their study all failed the "Sally-Anne" test, which tests the ability to understand that other people have thoughts and feelings that are not like one's own, referred to as Theory of Mind (Baron-Cohen, 1995). It is believed that this test is a central diagnostic criterion for ASD. Although the girls studied by Kopp and Gillberg (1992) understood the language of the test and the instructions, they were unable to think about other people's mental states. Nyden, Hjelmquist, and Gillberg (2000) also found that girls with ASD had a greater impairment with empathy and Theory of Mind skills. This suggests that girls with ASD have more difficulty understanding what others are thinking and predicting the behaviors of others.

Girls tend to be passive and internalized and do not exhibit the more typical acting-out behaviors observed in boys. Kopp and Gillberg (1992) reported, "Although girls meet the core deficits for a diagnosis, they do not have the same behavioral phenotype as boys. More often they would be diagnosed with a learning disorder or perceptual problems. Boys tend to be more aggressive and domineering and show strong initiative for their insistence on sameness. These behaviors make their problems much more difficult to ignore or dismiss" (p. 97).

Further, the diagnosis of ASD often focuses on language deficits, tantrums, and aggression. "These behaviors are all less common in girls than boys in the general population. Therefore, the relative rarity of girls with ASD may reflect a global difference between boys and girls rather than any factor that is specific to autism" (Smith, 1997, p. 2).

By Danielle (Mother of Mattie at age 3)

As I finish cleaning up the breakfast dishes on this quiet Saturday morning, my attention is drawn to the urgency in Mattie's little footsteps. She is busily scurrying up and down the stairs in desperate search of her many baby dolls. In what has become a recurring scene at our house, Mattie is once again extremely adamant about finding every doll before she will play. Sensing that she is not far from a meltdown, I assist her in the hunt. After the last doll has been found, she is finally able to enjoy some peace.

Watching her begin to play with her dolls, I find myself traveling back to my own childhood. My sister and I were only 13 months apart, and I can remember spending hours playing with our dolls. In imitating my mom taking care of our little sister, we would cuddle, feed, burp, and change our dolls. Occasionally, Mom would let us have one of our sister's diapers, which was a huge treat for us. This made our dolls appear to be even more realistic.

In stark contrast, Mattie's approach to doll play seems to be more like work than fun. There is such determination in her eyes as she lines up her dolls side by side in a perfectly uniform row. Once her dolls are placed in this systematic way, she covers them with blankets from head to toe. I watch her intently, as I desperately try to understand why she plays this way. Why is she covering their faces? I know they are not real, but doesn't she even process the connection that they may not be able to breathe? Why isn't she cuddling them? After all, Mattie has a little brother whom I feed, burp, and change. Why isn't she imitating me like I did with my mom?

That evening when I went into Mattie's room to kiss her goodnight, one of my questions was answered. As I peeled back the layers of blankets to find a warm, blushed face and peaceful little girl, I finally understood why she covered her dolls' faces. She herself slept all cocooned in her blankets, covered from head to toe. I wonder if the blankets protect her from the world she struggles so hard to figure out? Whatever the reason, I look forward to peeling back the covers every night and kissing her sweet face.

Pretend play is also different for girls. Pretend play may appear to be present, but it is deceiving. As Danielle observed in her daughter Mattie, what appeared to be pretend play was part of her stereotypical and rigid behaviors of ASD. Smith (1997) reports that girls play more than boys and engage in fewer stereotypical and repetitive play behaviors. Girls are observed as having more appropriate play skills (Lord, Schopler, & Revicki, 1982). Thus, girls with ASD may appear to engage in pretend play, but it is more rigid and ritualistic than the play of typically developing peers. Girls with ASD can perform complex doll play and even have imaginary friends similar to typically developing girls, but there is a qualitative impairment in their play – it often lacks reciprocity and is too controlling for typical girls (Attwood, 1999). According to Atwood, the dominance and intensity of play is out of the norm for a young girl. A highly trained clinician must closely examine pretend play for underlying rigid behaviors and atypical characteristics.

Characteristics Reported in Girls with ASD

- Good social imitation skills

- Low motor development

- Odd play skills

- Repetitive questioning

- Passive or lack of initiative

- Non-aggressive behaviors

- Attentional problems

- Disorganized or lack of focus

- Lack of empathy

- Difficulty understanding humor

(From Attwood, 1999; Kopp & Gillberg, 1992;
Lord et al., 1982; Smith, 1997)

What are the long-term indicators for a lack of diagnosing girls with ASD? According to Miller (2003), the under-diagnosing of women contributes to the marginalization of females on the spectrum. If we do not appropriately identify girls at an early age, women will continue to stay in the background and live in seclusion. "We have certain acceptable roles for women in our culture that provide a cover for women with ASD. Married women who stay at home do not have to deal with people in the outside world. Or a single woman who lives alone and keeps to herself does not draw public scrutiny. The lack of identification has a negative long term impact on women as adults. They continue to live in isolation" (Miller, 2003, p. xxii). Eustacia Cutler, mother of Temple Grandin, describes the isolation that is often felt among family members with children on the autism spectrum.

By Eustacia (Mother of Temple Grandin)

From *A Thorn in My Pocket* (2004)

I practice Bach on the piano. Temple, on the floor beside me, is absorbed in crumpling a newspaper. She squeezes it, watches it slowly spring open, shreds it, gazes at the pieces floating about her. I stop playing and try to entice her with colored plastic cups. She stares at them for a moment, then returns to her newspapers. Again, I tell myself that children have to find their own playthings, that I mustn't always be the one to instigate the game. Yet, she looks so forlorn, sitting there absorbed in her tattered plaything, sooty with newspaper ink, like a slum child nobody cares for. My pretty baby with her blue eyes and blonde curls, she who would prefer that I leave her alone. The calm, eerie snub cuts deep.

And so for today we each neglect the other. Isolated, numb, we play it safe: I in my world; she in hers. But what is her world? I turn back to the Bach. I'm not very good at it, but it's better than nothing. She hums. (p. 19)

In summary, our assessment tools are not designed to separate out the subtle differences in males versus females with ASD. Research on autism began more than 50 years ago by Dr. Leo Kanner (1943), who studied the classic characteristics of ASD. In subsequent years neither educational nor medical researchers have changed the diagnostic tools to reflect the wide spectrum of characteristics for boys and girls with ASD. Our current assessment tools for ASD do not examine the full range of symptoms, and thus do not detect gender differences. According to Attwood (1999), girls and boys have a similar profile, but girls have a less severe expression of the characteristics. Researchers must begin to vet out those slight differences and better train clinicians for diagnosing girls with ASD. Based on the ratio of boys to girls in autism, 4:1, and Asperger Syndrome, 10:1, it is our belief that girls with ASD are under-diagnosed and require special consideration and treatment.

The Diagnosis

By Jazz (age 16 with ASD)

My life is great because I'm not shunned by anyone. I can fit in just fine, with just about any group (well, except for the people who do the wrong things). People see me for who I am, and most people see me as a regular person. This is good, as I want people to accept me. My family can talk to me easily, and I am not isolated from anyone.

But it wasn't always like this. When I was 4 years old, I was diagnosed with autism. I used to bang my head against the wall, floor, anything I could spot. I also flailed, shrieked, bit, wouldn't look anyone in the eyes, and did just about everything else that children with autism do. Although I matured fast as a baby, I became mute at the end of my infant years, before I was 2 years old. Then, if I ever did talk, all I spoke was gibberish to the people who saw me. To put it in simpler terms, I was in what my mom called "the Void," which she describes as "my time in darkness."

Things were scary, like the fact that people "discarded" me and my mom out of the social realm, just because they thought that my mom didn't know how to control me. My autism was something that NEITHER of us could control at the time, and for that reason we were shunned by the people we knew. And, worse yet, the doctors who diagnosed me with autism said that I would likely never be able to speak English. They said that I might have to be put in some kind of home full of "people like me," who were also "misfits," and that if I was lucky I would get my high school diploma by the age of 21. They called me "mentally retarded," with my IQ at the time being 50. Had I understood what they said of me at the time, I most likely would have broken down and gone even further into "The Void." If my loving mom had not been as faithful as she is, she would have given up on my case and we might still be outcasts.

Jazz describes the early years of her diagnosis with ASD and its impact on the family. Receiving a diagnosis of autism or Asperger Syndrome can be devastating on one hand. On the other hand, it can be a blessing to finally have some answers. Coping with the diagnosis of ASD is unique for each family. Some families rejoice in knowing that finally there is a diagnosis while others go into denial. The stages of grief for a family when learning a child has a disability can include:

- Denial
  It can't be happening to us, to our family, to our daughter.

- Anger
  Why is this happening? It is unfair.

- Bargaining or Negotiating
  What can we do to change things, how can we cure this disability?

- Depression
  We can't do anything; nothing is working.

- Acceptance
  Everything has a purpose, and we can learn and grow from this experience.

Whatever your stage of grief, the following strategies will assist you and your family in creating a positive outcome after the diagnosis. Families and caregivers are often confused and overwhelmed after receiving a diagnosis of ASD. There are myriad questions and treatment options to consider. The following are some steps for sorting through this complex period.

- **Join a networking/support groups.** The best advice for a family new to ASD is to network with other families. ASD support groups exist in every state in the country. Start by contacting the local Autism Society of America (ASA) chapter or go to their national website [www.autism-society.org]. This organization was established in the early 1960s as a parent advocacy organization. It now has chapters throughout the United States. If ASA does not meet your needs, look to other parent support groups for children with disabilities. Your local school district can give you the name and phone number of parent education networks in your area.

Danielle and Barbie (Mothers)

We met each other in the psychologist's waiting room while our 5-year-old children were attending their weekly social skills group. Our friendship grew as we shared our experiences with our children and the many obstacles we faced. We agreed that when our children were first diagnosed, we didn't know where to go, who to call, or what to do with our newfound information. We realized that we had wasted much time, needless frustration, and many tears, on trying to research local resources to help our children. It was at this time that we decided to start a support group.

Our first meeting consisted of 15 parents. It was wonderful to be able to share stories, intervention ideas, and alternative therapy options with other people who were living in our same autism world. We made our community aware of the support group through word of mouth, Internet websites, e-mails, and flyers. We have just begun our fifth year and have grown to over 250 families.

- **Read everything on ASD accuracy and credibility.** Due to the rising attention to ASD, increasingly more companies target parents who are seeking a fast cure for ASD. Some of these companies' claims are not legitimate, so parents must be cautious. Consult your pediatrician, ask other parents, and use your own judgment when reading books, articles, and postings on the Internet.

- **Select appropriate treatments.** As parents receive the diagnosis of ASD, they often seek treatment options that will assist their daughter with ASD and its symptoms. There are many alternative and complementary treatments available. For example, auditory integration therapy, gluten- and casein-free diet, facilitated communication, and vitamin therapy. These treatments have not been scientifically proven to be effective for the ASD population. Focus on methods that have scientific evidence to support their effectiveness. The National Research Council (2001) has published *Educating Students with Autism* to assist parents and professionals in discerning the most appropriate interventions. Parents must take great care to determine what is appropriate for the unique needs of their daughter with ASD.

Questions to Ask When Reviewing the Literature and Other Information on Treatment Options

- Is there scientific evidence to prove effectiveness for children with ASD?

- Is the treatment safe for children?

- What are the costs? What are the side effects?

- How much training and family time is required?

- Is the treatment individualized to the child?

- What are the credentials of the organization or business that is promoting the treatment?

- Overall, what are your true feelings with regard to the treatment or method?

- **Take your time.** Although we know that early intervention is critical to positive outcomes for children with ASD, it is acceptable and appropriate to take your time to acknowledge the diagnosis and thoughtfully and systematically plan for the future. As parents and professionals are planning a comprehensive behavioral and educational intervention plan, do not attempt to implement every new therapy and complementary treatment at once. This can overwhelm both the child and the family. Prioritize the most scientifically effective methods and implement them consistently and systematically over time.

By Shirley (Grandparent of Haley, age 9)

My husband and I have taken on the roles as the main caregivers while their father is at work for our 9-year-old granddaughter, Haley, who has high-functioning autism, and her 8-year-old brother, Michael. Although we feel blessed to be a part of their lives, it is difficult at times to be solely responsible for their care. Our experience as parents, unfortunately, didn't prepare us for the hard work it takes to raise a grandchild with special needs. There are some days when I feel that I can't drive her to one more doctor, therapist, or social skills group. However, then I think about other families who are worse off than us, and that thought gets me through another day. We have been fortunate to find a local support group that has helped us to realize we are not alone in the autism journey. Networking with other families has provided us with information on interventions as well as friendships that otherwise may not have developed.

Conclusion

The current prevalence rates attest to the fact that we have an over-identification of males in special education, including ASD. Professionals in the medical and educational fields have limited their assessment of ASD to include the male-only characteristics of this disability. Females on the spectrum are not being identified for services at the same rate as their male counterparts primarily due to their more compliant behaviors and more passive roles.

There is no denying that when a young girl is identified with ASD, there is a profound effect on the lives of families. Although the diagnosis can be traumatic initially, it doesn't necessarily mean it's the end of the world. There are several proactive strategies that parents can take to cope with the diagnosis and plan for the future of their daughter.

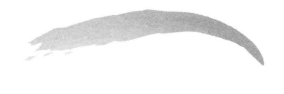

CHAPTER 2

The Early Years

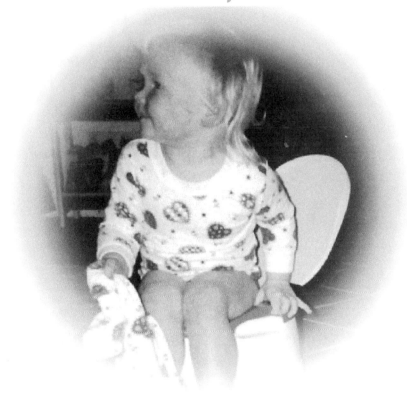

*I*n Chapter 1 we outlined some of the distinguishing characteristics of girls with ASD and explored some strategies for dealing with the diagnosis and moving forward. We will now examine some of the most practical techniques for addressing their individual needs, including behavioral problems, sleeping, toileting, and eating – major concerns in the home and community. We will also share insight from families and young women on the spectrum on their daily struggles and successes.

Tantrums and Tears

By Eustacia (Mother of Temple Grandin)

From *A Thorn in My Pocket* (2004)

Temple rips off her lilac flowered wallpaper in long jagged shreds, digs through her blue plastic crib mattress with its bunny rabbits, claws between the springs, pulls out the stuffing, flings it about, eats it, chews it, spits it in great gray wads. She goes into a spasm of giggling and spitting. I try to calm her; she scratches free and runs out the front door. In the middle of the road, our country road with the stone wall running along it, she yanks off her clothes, squats and poops. Again, I try to scoop her up. She laughs her crazy laugh and squirms from my arms.

Back in her own room, she tears up everything, throws every-thing — toys, clothes, pillows, wastepaper basket. But she throws them all in the same corner of the room. Is this some kind of organization, some intention, some target she has in mind? Am I the target? I toss the ball. She lets it bounce past her, poops again and smears her feces on the torn wallpaper. I repaper her room and fight despair.

The tantrums don't abate. Finally in a burst of my own rage, I pick up Temple, mid-scream, carry her flailing into her room, sit her down and close the door. Let her demolish the room if she likes; she'll have to do it alone. Almost as soon as I shut the door, she stops screaming. Is it no sport to have a tantrum with-out an audience? Or does she prefer to be alone? (p. 20)

This story reflects just some of the behavioral issues that may be exhibited by girls with ASD. Behavior meltdowns, tantrums, and constant arguing can occur in a variety of settings and can easily escalate if parents and professionals do not have a plan for decreasing problem behaviors and teaching appropriate skills. The following information applies to girls at any age. We are introducing this information early in the book so that you will have the skills during any period in your child's development.

Although girls with ASD often exhibit less aggressive behaviors than boys, most exhibit behaviors that can interfere with their ability to benefit from learning and be independent. Effective behavior intervention programs are often the most important element for a successful classroom or home environment. The following are important steps to developing a successful program. Each will be discussed further.

- Review the elements of a functional assessment – parents and professionals must determine why the behavior is occurring.
- Develop and write a behavior intervention plan for home and school.
- Identify and implement reinforcement techniques.
- Investigate environmental changes to support the behavior.
- Plan a reactive program – determine how to react to the problem behavior.
- Develop a crisis management plan.

Both parents and school personnel can develop a concrete plan for addressing problem behaviors. An effective program will focus on two main strategies (Ernsperger, 2003):

1. Proactive programming
2. Reactive programming

Principles of Proactive Programming vs. Reactive Programming

Problem behaviors do not change by implementing reactive strategies only. You cannot discipline away a behavior that is part of the child's disability. Instead, you must teach new replacement skills. Highly effective programs for girls with ASD should emphasize proactive strategies for reducing problem behaviors and teaching replacement skills. The following shows the major differences between proactive and reactive programming,

Proactive vs. Reactive Programming

Proactive	Reactive
Assumes the problem behavior serves a purpose for the child and is meeting his/her needs	Waits for the problem behavior to occur and then responds with punishment
Teaches alternative and replacement skills that serve the same function as the target behavior	Focuses on the consequences or disciplinary actions for the behavior
Identifies the function or purpose of the behavior (i.e., escape and avoid)	Reinforces the problem behavior by providing attention to the child when the behavior is exhibited
Modifies the antecedents to the behavior and environmental controls	Does not significantly or permanently change the problem behavior
Reviews the causes of the problem behavior as well as environmental and sensory concerns	Does not teach new skills

A comprehensive intervention program for girls with ASD will provide a careful balance of proactive and reactive practices. This involves conducting a thorough functional assessment and developing an appropriate behavior intervention plan. Parents and professionals must determine (a) why the behavior is occurring,

(b) what environmental changes need to be made, and (c) what specific behaviors need to be taught.

Functional Assessment Made Easy

The Individuals with Disabilities Act, IDEA, is the federal law that regulates special education in schools for all students with exceptional needs. Part of the regulations requires school district personnel and parents to conduct a functional assessment and write a behavior intervention plan for students whose behavior impedes their learning. The requirement is stated within the individualized education program (IEP) and is conducted by a multidisciplinary team. Although girls with ASD do not always exhibit acting-out or aggressive behaviors, their lack of friendships and an inability to communicate effectively with their peers do meet the requirements for conducting a functional assessment. Age-appropriate social and communication skills are part of the IEP. Parents should request a functional assessment and behavior plan for their children with ASD.

Although it may seem that conducting a functional assessment is the role of school personnel, parents play an important part in this process. A functional assessment and behavior plan is a joint effort between school and home. Conducting a functional assessment and writing a behavior plan will save you hours of stress and frustration in the long run. Plus, it will focus on teaching new and appropriate skills.

A thorough functional assessment is the first step in a proactive program. It begins the process of understanding the purpose of the child's behavior. "Why is she exhibiting this behavior?" and "What new behaviors should we be teaching?" The following story addresses these puzzling questions that most parents face.

By Danielle (Mother of Mattie at age 3)

As we arrive for yet another doctor's visit, I can't help but think of some of the questions that are frequently asked. "Mrs. Wendel, could you explain one of your daughter's meltdowns, or should I say 'fits of rage' as you stated in the 30-page questionnaire?" Why was that such a hard question for me to answer? Was it the way the doctor looked at me, first with concern, then disbelief that this blonde-haired, blue-eyed little girl could do such a thing? Maybe it was my own helplessness of not knowing what was wrong with my daughter, or the insecurity that plagued me from constantly being judged by others for the way I handled my daughter's behaviors.

Why couldn't she just have a "fit of rage" right here, right now, in the doctor's office? How would he handle it? I find myself smirking at that very thought. Within a few minutes, the doctor enters the room and introduces himself. He then makes a pleasant comment about my daughter's blonde hair and bright blue eyes. I glance over toward Mattie, who is sitting quietly at a large round table looking into a box of fresh crayons that were offered to her upon our arrival. Never fails. It looks like she's going to be on her best behavior while we are here.

Once again, I begin to describe one of Mattie's meltdowns in hopes that this doctor can help us. "As the Legos fly across the room at a speed only my husband could attempt, I notice Mattie is having one of her frequent meltdowns. She has thrown all her Legos around the room and is banging her head on the tile floor in the kitchen as if it's no harder than a pillow. Startled and half aware of what just happened, I try to calm her down by holding her tightly in my arms. She proceeds to pull her hair out by the handfuls as she tries to kick her way out of my grasp. I manage to drag her into her bedroom, where the carpet may be a safer place. I close the door behind me, as I take a minute to calm myself down. I hear her as she pulls the drawers from her dresser onto the floor and throws her clothes and toys around the room in complete rage. I attempt to go back in the room, but find that Mattie has positioned her feet against the door, holding it shut while kicking it and screaming.

After a few minutes, I am finally able to force myself into the room. I pull her tightly into my arms and hold her as if she is drowning and I can't let her go further into the water. The tighter I hold her, the calmer she becomes. I rock her back and forth trying to calm her, while telling her to relax. I speak barely above a whisper. After what seems like about two hours, she finally exhausts herself enough to fall sound asleep in my arms."

Step 1. Defining Target Behavior: What Is the Problem?

Define an observable and measurable target behavior. Clearly identify a problem behavior that needs to be addressed. The multidisciplinary team, which includes the parents, may choose to target a behavior that can be easily corrected before moving to more challenging behaviors. For example, getting dressed in the morning may be easier to address than expanding the child's diet to include vegetables. Targeting lesser behaviors may build success for the child and make changing more challenging behaviors easier.

Step 2. Gathering Information: How Often or for How Long Does the Behavior Occur?

Information on the frequency and duration of the behavior is collected through direct observation. Observations focus on the frequency, duration, and intensity of the problem behavior. Watch your daughter around the house or in the community to determine how often or for how long the target behavior occurs.

Analyzing the environment is another important step in the functional assessment process. Take a close look at the home or classroom environment to determine what might be causing the behavior to occur. Is the house/classroom orderly and without clutter? Is there a routine and schedule for each day? Is it posted? Is there a quiet area or a break area to get away from sensory stimuli? (See Appendix: Environmental Checklist.)

Physiological factors are the last area of data collection that may influence problem behaviors. Girls with ASD often have medical issues that can increase maladaptive behaviors. Physiological areas to be considered in a functional assessment include

- Diet and nutrition
- Sleep patterns and fatigue
- Medication side effects
- Undiagnosed illnesses

It is important to carefully consider how these variables might be influencing your daughter's behavior. If the child is not eating properly or is awake for several hours each night, the outcome will be irritability and an increase in problem behaviors. The team can effectively address these issues and reduce further problem behaviors by working with the parents in developing an appropriate sleeping and eating program for the student.

Step 3. Developing a Hypothesis: What Is the Team's Best Guess?

The third step in a functional assessment is to review the data and identify the function of the problem behavior. The function of problem behaviors varies with each child. The following are common functions:

- Escape/avoidance: *Hitting a sibling to escape eating dinner. Crawling under the desk to escape having to complete a math assignment.*

- Attention seeking: *Screaming at the grocery store so mom will pay attention. Yelling out a swear word in class so their peers will look at them and laugh.*

- Power/control: *Refusing to put on their shoes when told by the parent. Tearing apart their spelling list when the teacher directs them to get to work.*

- Communication: *Throwing the toothbrush on the ground because they lack the communication skills to explain to the parent that the toothpaste has too strong a flavor. Not completing an assignment in class because they lack the initiative to request assistance.*

- Stress/frustration: *Arguing with the parent when they drive a new route to school. Talking excessively about South American flags when going on a field trip.*

- Self-stimulation or sensory stimulation: *Rocking back and forth when waiting in line at the movie theater. Playing with their hair in class when there is a substitute teacher.*

The team examines the information collected and develops a written statement regarding the purpose of the behavior. This is called the *hypothesis statement.*

The following are examples of hypothesis statements:

- Waiting in the bank line takes too long for Robin, so she hits other people in line in order to *escape* waiting.

- Samantha refuses to complete her breakfast because she does not like the texture of the seat on the kitchen chair. She attempts to run out of the kitchen in order to get away from the *sensory* stimuli of the chair.

- When Stephanie goes to the bathroom, she screams for her mother because she gets *frustrated* when pulling up her pants and washing her hands.

Each statement identifies the problem behavior and the environment where it most likely will occur, and provides an "informed guess" as to the purpose of the behavior for the child.

By Danielle (Mother of Mattie at age 3)

My daughter Mattie was extremely verbal at an early age. At times, her choice of words was unacceptable, and words like "butthead" and "stupid" would just fly out of her mouth. It didn't matter what we tried, nothing could stop her. One day, I finally had enough. I told her that those words were dirty and that if she felt like she needed to say them, she would have to say them in the bathroom into the toilet and with the door closed. When she had finished saying her words, she would have to flush away those dirty words. At first, our water bill increased a bit from all the flushing, but without an audience and having to make all those trips to the bathroom, her choice of words soon became much cleaner.

Danielle and her family realized that Mattie was saying her "dirty words" for attention and decided to change their reaction to her inappropriate behavior. By removing their attention, Mattie decreased her problem behavior.

Step 4: Developing a Behavior Intervention Plan (BIP)

The behavioral intervention plan is a written document that includes:

- An operational definition of the target behavior
- A summary of the relevant data
- A written hypothesis statement stating the function of the behavior
- A list of modifications to the environment
- Teaching replacement or alternative behaviors
- Criteria or outcome evaluation
- Consequence strategies: crisis intervention plan and reactive program

If you are working with a school district, they should have a copy of a BIP. If not, a sample BIP is included in the Appendix.

An effective behavior intervention plan consists of two main components: *replacement skills to be taught* and *modifications to the environment*. To be effective, the replacement behavior must be as effective and powerful as the maladaptive behavior. For example, if a young girl is receiving attention from peers every time she lifts her dress up inappropriately, the team must teach a social replacement skill that has the same outcome. Other replacement behaviors include asking for assistance, playing with peers appropriately, and requesting a break in the schedule.

Maintain High Expectations

Do not allow autism to be an excuse for bad behavior. According to Temple Grandin and Simon Baron-Cohen (*The Unwritten Rules of Social Relationships*, 2005), parents should maintain high expectations for their children and not allow them to be rude. "My mother expected me to perform when it came to basic manners – she didn't view my autism as a reason to lower her expectations of me" (p. 219).

By Lynley (Mother of Jazz at age 3)

From *Autism Is Not a Life Sentence* (2006)

For me, as for many parents of children on the autism spectrum, going into public was a harrowing experience. Jessica was a toddler that was often hard to handle. I remember the days before I had children of my own, talking negatively about parents who put leashes and harnesses on their kids. I spoke with such self-righteous abandon about how such things were meant for dogs, and that if people couldn't control their children, perhaps they shouldn't have them at all. Ahhhh … the ignorance of youth.

I took Jessica to the grocery store one afternoon before her fourth birthday, out of necessity. I had to steer the cart with one hand and keep one arm around her to keep her in the cart. In the pickle and peanut butter aisle, she went berserk. She started with some gentle flapping and squealing to let me know she wanted to get out of the seat, and then she struck out at me and kicked and screamed. Her body went rigid, and she pushed upwards with her arms with such force that it nearly launched her little body out of the cart. When I grabbed her, she proceeded to bang her head against mine, and kick me with her legs. I knelt, to get better leverage on the floor, but the episode caught her so quickly, and the emotional storm blew in with such force, that it was just a few moments before I was lying with her in the floor, bracing her arms and legs, and taking the full blows of her head against my chin and chest to prevent her from hurting her head against the floor or the shelving. Not surprisingly, we drew a crowd of onlookers. After two or three minutes, the wildness in her eyes subsided, and I was finally able to release her. We were a mess. She had busted my bottom lip against my teeth with her head, and had my blood in her hair. I dug into my purse to get some tissues to clean up the tears and the blood, and the smeared mascara.

Then I put her back into the cart. I still had to get milk and eggs and detergent, and there was nobody to help me. I remember feeling angry. I was angry at the people who had watched helplessly as we endured that storm, and said nothing. I was angry at the lady in front of me at the checkout counter, who chatted with her seemingly normal toddler about his choice of breakfast cereal. I was angry because of the questioning looks from the manager in the glass booth at the customer service desk, as he surveyed me and the stains on my shirt from the floor of aisle #3 and the blood from my lip, then looked to my giggling and babbling filthy child in the cart, and her matted bloody mass of blonde hair on top. He exchanged a knowing

glance with the security officer, and that made me angrier.
What could anybody know about it? (p. 66)

This story is a perfect example of why parents need a behavior plan. This mother was clearly overwhelmed with the sudden outburst exhibited by her daughter. Although parents can often predict when outbursts will occur, many don't have a structured plan for how to prevent the behavior from occurring or appropriate steps for reacting when the problem behavior does occur. A behavior plan includes these important steps for parents to follow to reduce the anger and frustration that often comes with having a young girl with ASD.

Reinforcement Strategies

Since all human beings are motivated by positive reinforcement, reinforcement strategies are key elements in teaching girls with ASD. Most typically developing children are reinforced through task completion and teacher praise, but children with ASD may not be reinforced through these internalized methods. They often require external motivation to maximize their learning and increase adaptive behaviors. Therefore, parents and professionals must make a list of highly desired motivators when teaching new skills. These motivators will vary, but may include computer time, new books, time to watch TV, toys, or other special activities. Remember, high-quality reinforcement increases and maintains desired behaviors. In the following, Jana reminds us that we are never too old to earn reinforcement.

By Jana (age 27 with ASD)

Please initiate a rewards program – even for adults. My husband created a sticker program for me, and it works wonders. I earn stickers throughout the day by waking up on time, working my intended hours, and resolving various issues without having breakdowns. If I attend parties or family events, which are always extremely difficult for me, I have the opportunity to earn double stickers. My rewards are grown-up, and my husband calculates the sticker-to-prize ratio. For instance, I can exchange 100 stickers for a shopping spree or save stickers up for several pieces of jewelry. I've earned designer handbags, watches, books, shoes, and money. I may be the oldest woman on a sticker program, but it reminds me to stay focused on my goals.

Reinforce Immediately

When first teaching a new skill or desired behavior, reinforcement must be immediate and continuous to ensure the desired behavior is repeated. As the child progresses with a newly acquired skill or behavior, the reinforcement schedule is decreased and becomes more intermittent. An intermittent schedule is like a slot machine: The student receives a pay-off at different intervals, but does not know when the pay-off will occur.

Environmental Controls in Home and School

Although teaching replacement skills is an ongoing daily activity and an integral part of the BIP, environmental modifications to the home and school must also be addressed. Some typical modifications include:

- Creating a break area for the child to go to in order to calm down
- Decreasing the amount of clutter
- Developing and posting a daily schedule
- Identifying specific age-appropriate rules and posting visual reminders
- Reviewing the sensory needs of the child and creating sensory activities (see p. 104)

Maintaining a calm and supportive environment will help to decrease problem behaviors. Most girls with ASD improve their behavior if their environment is predictable and meets their sensory needs. For example, most girls can effectively maintain appropriate behavior if the teacher has posted a visual schedule that is followed systematically and if sensory breaks are part of the schedule that include a variety of sensory activities that meet the student's needs.

Reactive Programming

Although the focus of a BIP should be proactive, it is also essential to develop a reactive program. Proactive programs focus on changing the environment, identifying sensory needs, and teaching replacement skills while reactive programs focus on the inappropriate behaviors after they occur. In a reactive plan, parents and professionals determine the steps that will occur after the child exhibits the maladaptive or problem behavior. For example, when Jessica from our story begins to tantrum in the grocery store, her mother needs a plan for how she will react to inappropriate behavior. Reactive programming can further decrease the frequency of problem behaviors and may help regain control in a crisis.

In a well-designed behavior program, reactive procedures are used minimally, and then only with respect for girls with ASD. Parents and professionals should be careful to not focus only on the inappropriate behaviors but adequately plan for proactive strategies.

By Danielle (Mother of Mattie at age 10)

As Mattie was maturing, I felt it was necessary to create some kind of a subtle cue that would let her know whether or not her behavior was appropriate. I started by simply saying, "Cool, Mattie" when she did something appropriate and "Not Cool" when she was displaying inappropriate behaviors. After a while, we graduated to nonverbal cues such as thumbs-up and thumbs-down, which were more age-appropriate. I can't believe how successful this was. By not bringing attention to the situation, she felt more in control of her behavior. Mattie loves the thumbs-up signal best.

Danielle created a reactive program for Mattie using a verbal reminder and a visual cue for when her behavior was inappropriate. Instead of reprimanding Mattie and calling too much attention to the inappropriate behavior, her mom gave her a thumbs-down as a gentle reminder.

Several strategies are available to address behaviors after they have occurred. The home and school team should consider the least intrusive methods for decreasing the likelihood of problem behaviors. Response cost, extinction, time-out, and crisis management are a few reactive techniques that may be used in the home and at school. These will all be discussed further in the following.

Response Cost

A response cost program is designed to remove a reinforcer when the problem behavior occurs. A response cost program is often used in conjunction with a token economy system. A token economy system is a proactive program that reinforces the appropriately displayed behaviors with a simple token (i.e., sticker, marble, or coin). Token economy systems can be implemented in a variety of settings and address many behaviors.

A response cost system is the removal of the token for an inappropriately displayed behavior. For example, the child may be highly reinforced by working on the computer. Therefore, the teacher has laminated the eight letters of the word "computer" and placed each letter on the child's desk. Each time the child exhibits the problem behavior, one letter is removed from the word "computer." For every letter that remains at the end of the day, the child receives 5 minutes of computer time – a highly favored activity.

Other response cost programs include point systems or removal of marbles from a jar. Response cost systems should be used cautiously because they can create anxiety within the child if a token is removed. Also, response cost systems do not teach replacement skills; they focus only on the consequence of the problem behavior. Therefore, it is necessary to teach the appropriate replacement skill for the inappropriate behavior and use reinforcement techniques.

Extinction

Extinction refers to the gradual decrease of the problem behavior as reinforcement is discontinued. Extinction attempts to reduce the problem behavior by eliminating the social reinforcement, or attention, that maintains the behavior. Many parents and teachers try to use "planned ignoring" to extinguish a child's problem behavior. Success depends on the function of the behavior and the ability of the adult to eliminate social reinforcement. If the function of the behavior is attention, it is imperative to remove all attention from the child. For example, even if the adults withhold attention, a child who screams and tantrums for attention may still have her needs met if she receives attention from the other students. Attention from everybody must be removed before planned ignoring will extinguish, or stop, the problem behavior.

Ignoring or paying little attention to problem behaviors can be used effectively with girls with ASD. However, it is important not to ignore self-injurious behaviors and aggression because of the likelihood the behavior will escalate. In some cases, parents and professionals must provide some minimal attention in order to secure the environment for the child and others.

Minimal attention includes:
- A calm and neutral voice
- Little or no eye contact
- Minimal physical restraint. Most states have very specific regulations for physically restraining students, and school personnel must use caution before any planned physical contact with a student.
- Reduced demands

Extinction is a planned reactive intervention and should be used only when the function of the behavior is reinforced through attention from others.

Time-Out from Reinforcement

Time-out means that the child receives no reinforcement. In the case of a typically developing child, being removed to an isolated area of the home or school may be considered time-out from reinforcement. However, this is generally not the case for girls with ASD, who will most likely perceive the time-out area as reinforcing because:

- No demands are being placed on them.
- The function of the behavior is often escape and avoidance.
- They can initiate self-stimulatory behaviors, which are highly reinforcing.
- They may require a break or quiet time.

Time-out from reinforcement must be carefully planned and used with caution to avoid reinforcing and increasing the problem behavior. For example, some students will continue to exhibit the inappropriate behavior in order to go to time-out area and thereby avoid school work.

Crisis Management

Despite careful planning and the development of proactive programming, parents and teachers are occasionally faced with a crisis. Individuals with ASD may experience a variety of stressors throughout their day, which may include a change in the schedule, losing a school assignment, or teasing from other students. These stressors can create a crisis situation if parents and school personnel are not detecting the early signs of stress for the child. Myles and Southwick (2005) refer to these early signs of stress as the rumbling stage. During the rumbling stage, the child may exhibit behaviors such as mumbling to herself, pacing back and forth, or tapping her fingers. Walker, Colvin, and Ramsey (1995) refer to this as Phase 2 of the crisis cycle, or the trigger (see p. 52).

Parents and professionals must be very aware of the specific triggers for each child. Problem behaviors can be most easily redirected or changed at the earliest point in the crisis cycle. Therefore, once a trigger has occurred for the child, it is important that appropriate and meaningful strategies be implemented to redirect the child to a preferred task. Encourage the use of previously taught replacement skills such as requesting a break or seeking assistance from a friend. Also, provide reinforcement if the child remains calm and follows simple directions. Positive reinforcement can diffuse this stage of the crisis cycle.

Crisis Cycle

Phase 1.   Calm; optimal; comfortable level; baseline
Student is competently and quietly working on school work.

Phase 2.   Trigger
Student accidentally breaks pencil and does not ask for assistance.

Phase 3.   Irritable; frustrated; demanding; anxious
Teacher tells the student to "get to work" and "stop daydreaming."

Phase 4.   Peak; chaos; tantrums
Student becomes anxious and upset with the teacher for not providing assistance and tears up her paper.

Phase 5.   De-escalation
Student starts drawing a picture of horses to calm down.

Phase 6.   Recovery
Teacher gives the student a new worksheet and pencil; student returns to work.

Based on Walker et al. (1995).

As we can see from the various phases of the crisis cycle, if early triggers are not addressed, the child will eventually move into Phase 4 or peak crisis. Myles and Southwick (2005) refer to this as the rage stage. If a child is in crisis, be sure to control your own responses. It is important for the adults to stay calm and reduce any signs that they are agitated or stressed. Refer to the strategies for extinction of a behavior.

A crisis team may be assigned to work with the child if a crisis occurs in school. The team should have a written plan that addresses the steps for diffusing the crisis and assisting the child in repairing the situation and returning to class. In the home, parents can write out a crisis plan. It is especially important for parents to have a written and supportive plan for addressing the crisis cycle. Parents need to be sure they have determined appropriate house rules, provided consistent follow-through, and maintained a neutral position.

The final stage of the crisis cycle is recovery. As with any crisis situation, the adults and the child may be exhausted and require a quiet break (Myles & Southwick, 2005). Minimal demands should be placed on the child during this time. The child should be directed to review her schedule and be given a simple task to complete while she recovers. This is not the time to discuss punishment or restitution because that can create another crisis situation. Wait an appropriate length of time, maybe a few hours, before determining the consequences for the actions.

A functional assessment and behavior intervention plan should not only be a part of the child's IEP but should also be developed for the home. Parents can write out a short plan for addressing problem behaviors utilizing both proactive and reactive programming. The behavior intervention program should focus on teaching replacement skills and reinforcing appropriately displayed behaviors. Again, reactive programming should occupy only a small portion of the overall behavior program for students with

ASD. These procedures are only considered after other strategies have failed. If crises continue to occur, it is time to reevaluate and reassess to determine the function of the behavior. Because many maladaptive behaviors are chronic, it may take the school team and parents many months to effectively teach a new skill. For example, a young girl may decrease her tantrums from seven times per day to four times per day. Therefore, it is important to focus on the process and celebrate the small changes.

Mr. Sandman

By Sue (Mother of Jamie, age 5)

Since my 5-year-old daughter, Jamie, was an infant, she never had problems going to sleep at night. In fact, bedtime at our house was usually uneventful. It wasn't until Jamie began attending school that we started having trouble putting her to bed. Most evenings still found her stressed from her school day, and she began having a hard time relaxing enough to be able to fall asleep within a reasonable timeframe. Strangely enough, exactly one hour after she finally fell asleep, she would wake up completely drenched in sweat and crying that she had a nightmare. It got to the point where I could set my watch by this nightly event. Because I didn't know what caused this behavior, I didn't know how to help her overcome it.

I started to worry when Jamie began to wake up every morning looking just as tired as when she went to bed the night before. Instead of getting up refreshed and ready to start a new day, she'd awaken with dark circles under her eyes and in an irritable mood.

Shortly after we changed her bed from a junior style with side rails to a big-girl bed, I began quietly slipping into her room several times during the night to make sure she hadn't fallen out of bed. It seemed that no matter what time of the night it was, she would look up at me and say, "Hi, mom." That's when I finally realized why she looked so exhausted every morning. She wasn't sleeping at night!

Sleep deprivation is a problem facing many families with children on the spectrum. For a variety of reasons, sleep patterns may become disrupted for you and your child. A lack of sleep creates stress for both the parents and the child with ASD.

When sleep is disrupted or when an individual does not get enough sleep, the result is often mood changes and poor problem solving. Sleep deprivation is often accompanied by increased cortisol levels (Hoffman, Sweeney, Gilliam, & Lopez-Wagner, 2006), our stress hormones. Therefore, sleep deprivation can create increased anxiety, aggressive behaviors, and poor adaptability. Both parents and professional agree that adequate sleep is required for maintaining focus, learning new skills, and increasing school performance (Weissbluth, 1999). The good news is we can create a sleep training program to address these issues.

It is important to understand that falling asleep and staying asleep are learned behaviors. We have to teach these skills to our children. Most children can be taught to go to sleep and stay asleep. As parents, we must carefully observe our children for signs of tiredness and put them to bed as soon as those signs are displayed.

Never Wait to Put a Child to Bed!

Parents often miss the subtle first signs of sleepiness and attempt to put their daughter to bed after she is too tired. Waiting to put a child to bed only creates hypersensitivity to the environment and a wired state of arousal. When the child is overly tired, the family experiences more stress and difficulty in putting the child to bed. Carefully observe the child for signs of tiredness such as irritableness, rubbing eyes, and whining. Create a bedtime routine that will result in the child being in bed prior to this time (Crowder, 2002).

Before starting any sleep training program, seek counsel from your pediatrician. Be sure to rule out any physical reasons why your daughter is not sleeping. Certain medications may cause insomnia, for example. If your pediatrician wants to prescribe a sleeping aid, be sure you fully understand the side effects.

Developing a Sleep Program

Parents must make a serious commitment to a sleep training program for it to be effective. If parents or other significant family members disagree or are not ready to implement the plan, it will have little chance of success. There are many things a family can do to create a positive sleep environment for their daughter with ASD, including (a) creating a soothing environment to meet the child's sensory needs, (b) developing a consistent schedule and routine for bedtime, and (c) establishing a few simple rules for the child to follow each night.

By Myron (Father of Mattie, age 11)

"Daddy, let's bug" is a common request around our house in the evening. My kids love for me to roll around on the carpet in the living room hugging and squeezing them. This started when our children were just babies. Mattie, especially, craved the deep pressure and the comfort it gave her. I could almost feel her relax within minutes of us playing this game. Over the years, I have come to enjoy "bugging" as much as my kids, and now I'm the one to propose, "let's bug."

The Bedtime Environment

The bedtime environment should support the child's sensory needs. Mattie enjoys "bugging" with her dad because it helps calm her sensory system before bedtime. Many girls with ASD have problems with sensory integration. Transitioning to bedtime often creates sensory arousal or hypersensitivity. The changes from daytime to nighttime, from daytime clothes to pajamas, and from movement to staying still can have a significant impact on the sensory system.

Parents and caregivers must observe the bedtime environment and be sure it addresses the sensory needs of the child. Consider the following sensory activities for bedtime:

1. Weighted blankets
2. Aromatherapy – especially lavender and vanilla because they are soothing

3. Dimming the lights
4. Rocking in a chair
5. Soft music – rhythmically, slow paced
6. More or less physical contact – depending on the child's needs
7. For older girls, teach a sequence of relaxation exercises through deep breathing and progressive muscle relaxation, which includes identifying a specific muscle and tightening and relaxing that muscle for a few seconds. For example, make a fist with your hand and hold for a few seconds, then relax the hand.

Sensory activities that are calming to the sensory system will help your daughter regulate her sensory system and be better able to make the adjustments and changes in her routine from day to night.

Schedules and Routines

The second component of a sleep program targets the bedtime schedules and routines. As mentioned earlier, all children demonstrate early warning signs of tiredness and should be put to bed immediately when these appear. The bedtime routine should be developed so that it ends at this time and does not extend the bedtime (Pantley, 2005).

For the plan to be successful, parents should select a series of specific activities that will always occur prior to bedtime and result in the child being in bed at the designated time. The activities may consist of the following:

1. Eat a light snack
2. Take a bath

3. Put on pajamas

4. Brush teeth

5. Read a story

6.. Cuddle

7. Say goodnight

A picture schedule provides a concrete visualization of the bedtime routine, allowing the child to focus on the important concepts for each step in the process. This, in turn, will assist in decreasing anxiety and making the bedtime environment less stressful. A picture schedule may be easily created for any situation as follows:

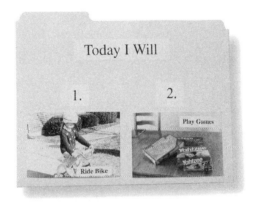

1. Select a heavy folder or clipboard.

2. Copy pictures of each of the activities (see above).

3. Velcro the pictures to the folder/clipboard.

4. Tape an empty envelope to the back of the folder/clipboard.

5. As each activity is finished, place completed pictures of each activity in the envelope.

6. Review each step with your daughter.

A timer may also be used for the bedtime schedule. Many children with ASD do not adequately understand the concept of time without a concrete representation. Timetimers® (www.timetimer.com)

are extremely effective in demonstrating to the child in a visual and concrete manner how much time is left, in this case, until bedtime.

Transition Toy

Select a toy or doll that is only associated with bedtime and relaxation. Keep this item in the bedroom. The toy or doll is only used when the child is in the bed and represents resting and sleeping. It is another visual reminder of bedtime.

Bedtime Rules

The third component of the sleep program is the writing and posting of bedtime rules. Because girls with ASD tend to be rule followers, it is helpful to write and post rules where your daughter can easily observe them in her bedroom. The rules would consist of staying in bed, keeping quiet, and not disrupting the house after being put to bed. Of course, the rules should be flexible enough to meet the needs of your daughter. For example, she may feel more comfortable sleeping in her bathing suit or sleeping under her bed in a sleeping bag or in her bed under the covers in her pajamas. This type of flexibility should be allowed if your daughter keeps within the stated boundaries and if otherwise considered appropriate. This decision may be based on the age and ability level of the child.

Night-Time Emergency Bag

Put a few key items in a canvas bag and place it next to your daughter's bed. The items may consist of a flashlight, a book, a fidget toy, or a bottle of water. Explain that these items are only for emergencies when the child wakes up early or wakes in the middle of the night. The purpose of the Night-Time Emergency Bag is to provide comfort items to your daughter so that she can calm herself down and return to sleep independently.

The sleep training program should be reviewed repeatedly with the child. Teaching good sleep habits will lead to a more adaptable and flexible child with less anxiety and mood swings, not to mention the benefits to parents and the whole family.

Bumps in the Night-Time Plan

Every sleep training program runs into problems along the way. Girls with ASD will experience changes in early childhood that may disrupt their sleep. The routine may be disrupted during illness, holidays, and vacations. Your daughter may also begin waking in the middle of the night if her circadian rhythms change as she grows older (Gurian, 2002). The circadian rhythm is a person's internal body clock that regulates the sleep cycle. Many factors can disrupt this cycle, such as traveling across time zones, exposure to light, changes in temperature and altitude, as well as hormonal changes.

When a child wakes in the middle of the night:
1. Keep the lights to a minimum.
2. Do not speak, or speak as little as possible.

3. Decrease all interactions, including hugs and kisses.

4. Give your daughter her Night-Time Emergency Bag and let her learn to put herself back to sleep.

Some parents decide to put locks on their daughter's bedroom door for safety. This is an important decision, and parents should consider several options prior to installing a lock on the door. For example, a locked door may prevent the child from gaining access to the bathroom, seeking help in the middle of the night, or escaping the house in case of an emergency. If you are concerned that your daughter is roaming the house or leaving the house in the middle of the night, a lock may be needed, at least temporarily, for safety reasons.

When temporary changes occur in the sleep program, be sure to return to the bedtime plan as quickly as possible. While good sleeping habits can be learned, so can bad sleeping habits (Murkoff, Eisenberg, & Hathaway, 2003). Be prepared to stick to the routine throughout her childhood and adolescence. Your daughter will not outgrow the need for good sleeping habits. The specifics of the schedule and the pre-bedtime activities may change, but a structure must always be in place to support sufficient sleep.

By Valija (Mother of Madelyn, age 10*)*

I wish that I could take my daughter in my arms and hold her, love her, kiss her, and squeeze her ... but she gets frustrated when I come into her space without asking. It's extremely hard as a parent not to be able to hug your child when you want to, but I respect my daughter's space and try my best to be understanding. Although it can be very hard at times, I am thankful when she lets me kiss her goodnight!

To Sleep, Perchance to Dream ...

If you have a daughter with ASD who is experiencing sleep difficulties, chances are that you are sleep deprived, too. Sleep deprivation is extremely exhausting and can create a large amount of stress in the home. It is important for parents to assess their own sleep needs and create a sleep program for themselves. Seek medical advice if you are experiencing sleep difficulties. A comprehensive sleep program will assist the entire family in reducing stress and providing for a more relaxed environment.

No More Diapers!

By Lynley (Mother of Jazz, age 16)

Toilet-training Jazz was difficult; we worked on it for over two years. However, her ability to toilet-train became a good indication of the effectiveness of using a trigger. What I mean is that if you use "whatever works" for the child in helping to shape behavior, it will start happening a lot faster. It was impossible to know whether or not Jazz responded to prompts via food reward, as in "let's use the potty and if you tinkle in the potty, I will give you ice cream," or something similar. It would only work if she was hungry, and often she was completely uninterested.

I tell parents to ask themselves what it is that their child really WANTS to have, to do, to eat, and then start to play around with those things as an incentive. What Jazz really wanted was to watch her videos. I had tried everything from offering

63

more story time, all kinds of food rewards, to toys and games and songs. With each new pursuit of the ultimate trigger, my attempt always seemed like a failure. However, my perception is different in that most others don't accept failure. Each time I found that there was a method or a reward that was ineffective, I considered it a small victory, because I had succeeded in discovering something that did not work. I had eliminated one more possibility on the way to finding the one probability!

At long last, I took every single one of the videos out of her room and boxed them up. Jazz was very agitated about this, but I made it clear that what she had to do to watch a video was go to the potty. When she did, she was allowed to earn a video back. When she had an accident, all the videos she had earned disappeared, and she started over again. I didn't use an angry voice, but I was firm with her, even through the screaming and inevitable meltdowns. It was difficult on me. We all sympathize with the urge to give in to a screaming child, but I kept thinking that a little difficulty on the front end would prevent a much larger difficulty for everyone later on.

Jazz was toilet-trained in two weeks' time. No more accidents or wet beds, and perhaps best of all, NO MORE DIAPERS! It was worth the two weeks of screaming and melting down to achieve this freedom.

Toileting a young girl with ASD can be challenging. Researchers suggest that girls are often toilet-trained 3-5 months earlier than boys, but this may be different for girls with ASD (Pantley, 2007), whose developmental delays in speech, motor skills, and problem solving can interfere with the toilet-training process. There are many excellent resources for toilet training (see Resources in the Appendix).

The following guidelines are created to address the specific needs of girls with ASD that are not addressed in the mainstream literature. First, we will examine some of the readiness skills required for toilet-training.

Is It the Right Time?

When deciding if it is the right time for toilet-training, several prerequisite skills must be considered: physical readiness, social readiness, sensory readiness, and overall family readiness.

Physical readiness for toilet-training involves muscle control (Krueger, 2001). Notice if your daughter can stay dry for one to two hours. Also, consider whether your daughter has adequate muscle control for her daily activities. Observe whether she is coordinated in her play and if she has good motor skills. Simple dressing skills should also be present, such as pulling on shirts and pants. If she has tight muscles and can stay dry for longer periods of time, she might be ready for toilet-training.

Social readiness is also important for toilet-training. Some girls may not appear to be interested in using the toilet. Your daughter may seem socially aloof and may not want to model mommy using the restroom. Read your daughter's social clues and determine if she seems interested in imitating others in the restroom. You might have to use some of the positive incentives that were tried by Lynley Summers in our story.

By Shirley (Grandparent of Haley at age 6)

My granddaughter Haley never liked sitting on the potty chair, and when we tried the big toilet, the flushing scared her. At school, she would only go to the restroom with another classmate. This was so the classmate could make sure that no one would flush while Haley was using the restroom.

I still remember taking a family trip to Disneyland when Haley was 6 years old. We stood in the line at the ladies' restroom for what seemed like hours. When we finally reached the front of the line, Haley started screaming and thrashing around trying to get out of my arms. When I managed to get her into the stall, I told her that I would trick the automatic flush and reassured her that it would not flush while she was on. This trick worked, and to this day we still trick the auto flush.

Sensory readiness is also important. As mentioned earlier, the sensory system of girls with ASD is often heightened, which means they can be easily overwhelmed with the many sights, sounds, and smells in the bathroom. Like Haley above, your daughter may appear to be scared of the flushing noises from the toilet. Or she may be overly sensitive to the smells. Additionally, the kind of underwear you select may be causing sensory problems. Some girls with ASD experience tactile defensiveness to certain textures of materials. Frilly underwear or underwear with seams in the crotch may cause irritation, and the child may refuse to wear them. These sensitivities can impact the outcome of a toileting program.

Consider the following activities for calming the sensory system when using the bathroom:

- Use a weighted lap belt or shoulder belt; small blankets or long socks filled with heavy materials such as rice, beans, or ankle weights.

- Rock or bounce on an exercise ball.
- Play soft music in the restroom to calm the auditory system.
- Put a dimmer switch on the bathroom lights.
- Select underwear with no lace, no tags, and no seams.

The sensory system should be adequately addressed before the child can successfully use the toilet.

Finally, *family readiness* plays an important role in toilet-training. A toileting program is a family affair and must be consistently implemented by all family members. Therefore, a toileting program should only be initiated when the household is calm. During the early years, most families of girls with ASD are going through medical evaluations and other testing situations. These outside influences can create a lot of stress. Therefore, it may be better to wait to implement a toileting program until things have settled down.

Many typically developing children initiate using the toilet by expressing an interest and by imitating their parents or siblings (Pantley, 2007). Individuals with ASD are often delayed in their imitation skills and may not attempt to imitate their parents. Some children may verbally request to sit on the toilet. For girls with ASD, their expressive skills (talking) may be delayed. Therefore, they may not ask to use the toilet or show any interest in the bathroom, even though they are otherwise ready for toilet-training. Keep in mind, receptive skills tend to be more advanced in girls with ASD, which means they can understand much more than they can express or explain in words. To check your daughter's receptive skills, see if she can follow two-step simple directions; for example, "go in your room and get your pants." If she has the receptive skills, she may be ready for toilet-training.

Getting Started

Once you have decided it is time to get started, you have some serious questions to consider: How often should I take her? What kind of potty chairs should we use? What about use of reinforcement? These are all valid concerns. Also, a few components of a structured toileting program must be in place, as discussed below.

Scheduling

First, girls with ASD need a structured schedule for toileting. Girls with ASD tend to be visual learners and will be more successful with a picture schedule of what is expected. The visual checklist may include pictures of the following:

1. Walk into the bathroom.
2. Pull down panties.
3. Hold handles and sit on the toilet.
4. Go pee.
5. Take toilet paper.
6. Wipe private area.
7. Stand up and pull up pants.
8. Flush toilet.
9. Wash hands.
10. Dry hands and exit.

After the schedule has been developed and posted, it is important to practice each step. Your daughter can practice several times throughout the day and should be praised for following each step even if she does not urinate on the toilet. The goal is for the toileting schedule to be a positive activity.

Another visual strategy to support the toileting plan is to copy several pictures of the toilet and place them around the house and in the car. Due to a delay in expressive language, some girls with ASD have difficulty asking to go to the toilet. The pictures of the toilet are to be used as a way for her to communicate her need to toilet. Watch for clues that she may need to use the restroom, offer her the toilet picture, and say "It looks like you need the toilet." Then walk her to the toilet and have her follow the visual steps. Visual pictures will assist her in using the toilet.

Lastly, there are many wonderful books and videos for children on toilet-training. These resources can be helpful in teaching the new vocabulary and in explaining to young children why they use the toilet and what happens when they get to the toilet. Pretend play is another way to assist the child in learning about toilet-training. Using favorite dolls and stuffed animals as role models for using the toilet is another visual support.

Selecting a Potty Chair

Once the picture schedules and pictures of the toilet are developed, it is time to select a potty chair. When doing so, consider the following basic requirements:

- The base is safe and secure.
- A foot rest is provided.

- It fits the child's physique.
- It has side rails for stability (Wolraich, 2003).

Also, if you have more than one toilet in the house, be sure to practice on all of them. Girls with ASD can become rigid and may begin to prefer only one toilet. Support your daughter in being flexible and use a variety of toilets at home and in the community.

Using Reinforcement

Lynley's story emphasizes the importance of not giving up on toilet-training. She was able to keep positive while finding a motivator that worked for her daughter. Jazz learned quickly that by using the potty she would be rewarded with a video.

The use of reinforcers for successful toileting varies. Some families believe that positive praise and enthusiasm are enough to create a successful outcome. Other families have chosen to use candy, stickers, or favorite activities for rewards for successful toileting. If your daughter does not appear to be motivated to use the toilet, it might be effective to use some tangible reinforcement. Examples of reinforcement include small candies (M&Ms), a favorite sticker, or a few minutes of watching a favorite video.

In the beginning, it is important to reinforce the child for each close approximation to using the toilet. If she walks into the bathroom and sits on the toilet – even without success – reinforce her attempt. After she has made several positive attempts, fade the reinforcement with each attempt until you are only providing positive verbal praise. On a cautionary note, if the child has an accident, do not punish her by removing the reinforcement. Just simply clean up in a calm manner and try again later.

Some young girls with ASD experience constipation in the early years. This may be due to poor diet, insufficient fluid intake, or fear of having a bowel movement. If you notice that the stool is hard or infrequent, or if it is painful for your daughter to have a bowel movement, consult with your pediatrician. Most constipation can be treated with dietary changes, such as:

- Increase fluids, including juices.
- Increase fiber, including foods such as baked beans, refried beans, spaghetti and meatballs, vegetable soups, broccoli, and raisins.
- Check side effects of any medications.
- Consult with your physician when using over-the-counter products such as laxatives and suppositories.
- Review behavior management strategies. If you daughter has experienced painful bowel movements, she may hold her stool, which can cause constipation. Be sure to encourage sitting on the toilet for a few minutes each day and reward her for success (Krueger, 2001).

Chronic constipation can cause encopresis, which is long-term fecal impact and soiling, resulting in accidental bowel movements and leaking of the bowel. Early and ongoing treatment for constipation will result in a healthy digestive system. Therefore, if you suspect or notice any sign of constipation, please consult your family physician or pediatrician.

Is It the Wrong Time?

After reviewing the list of readiness skills, you may conclude that it is not the right time to start a toilet-training program. Keep in mind, you cannot coerce or force a child to use the toilet. It is more appropriate to wait and have a successful outcome than to push the child. Be careful not to use even subtle statements, such as "Big girls go on the potty" or "All your friends are using big girl panties." Such statements can create an unwanted power struggle, which can create serious long-term problems.

There is not one universal toilet-training program that is effective for all children. Review the literature and consult a developmental pediatrician to determine the best plan for the individual child. If it is not the right time, take a break for a few months. Let your daughter know it is not her fault that toilet-training is not progressing smoothly. Return to diapers for a short period. It is not uncommon for girls with ASD to experience stress, anxiety, and a lack of concentration in the early years. It is better to wait for her and you to be ready. At the same time, it is critical for the child to become toilet-trained at a reasonable age for countless reasons, including independent functioning and fitting in with the peer group.

Just Take a Bite

By Jana (age 27 with ASD)

My appetite is ever shifting. As a baby, I ate my fair share of bugs, dog food, and dust bunnies. As a tot, nothing was inedible. Then something changed. I recall gagging on bananas, mashed potatoes, vitamins, and yogurt. My mother would find enormous wads of my partially dissolved vitamins in the wastebasket. Finger food became my enemy, and I struggled to keep from throwing up while examining others' eating habits.

Sharing a meal with family and friends can be a rewarding and life-affirming activity. There is nothing more satisfying than a lazy morning brunch, a picnic in the park, celebrating with holiday treats, or having lunch with friends in the school cafeteria. Eating and sharing a meal is a wonderful experience – unless you are a resistant eater or you have a resistant eater in your family. Then eating and mealtimes are often stressful, chaotic, and involve constant negotiation. Mealtimes and celebrations can soon turn disappointing due to unfulfilled expectations and dashed hopes when a resistant eater refuses to share a meal with family and friends.

While it is difficult to estimate the number of girls on the autism spectrum who experience food aversions and eating challenges, many girls, like Jana, struggle with eating challenges. According to Mayes and Calhoun (1999), 75% of children diagnosed with ASD experience atypical feeding patterns and have limited food preferences. Approximately half of the individuals with autism studied were hypersensitive to textures and lumps in the food.

Further research on resistant eating was conducted by Wing (2001), who reported that nearly two-thirds of the 230 children with ASD in her clinic experienced resistance to food, which included limited food diets and severe food fads. As represented by the research, the numbers of individuals with ASD who struggle with eating a balanced and appropriate diet is overwhelming.*

Who Are Resistant Eaters?

Resistant eaters are a mixed group of boys and girls who have food aversions.

Some eaters have medical issues or physical impairments, while others have a sensory integration dysfunction or poor oral-motor skills. Oral-motor skills include age-appropriate tongue control, chewing, and swallowing skills. There is not one single characteristic that identifies resistant eaters. For our purposes, the term "resistant eater" applies to any girl with ASD who meets the following characteristics.

Characteristics of a Resistant Eater

Resistant eaters often exhibit one or more of the following:
1. Limited food selection. Total of 20 foods or fewer.
2. Limited food groups. Refuses one or more food groups.
3. Anxiety and/or tantrums when presented with new foods. Gags or becomes ill when presented with new foods.
4. Food jags. Requires one or more foods be present at every meal prepared in the same manner.
5. Diagnosed with a developmental delay such as autism, Asperger Syndrome, or pervasive developmental disorders-not otherwise specified.

---

*The following treatment strategies for addressing resistant eaters are excerpts from *Just Take a Bite* (Ernsperger & Stegen-Hanson, 2004). Used with permission.

A thorough review of the young girl's medical history and assessment of oral-motor delays by trained professionals is necessary before beginning a treatment program.

A collaborative team approach to assessment and treatment ensures that a written plan is implemented across settings and throughout the child's day.

A Comprehensive Treatment Plan

Solving the mealtime dilemma is not a quick fix. In most situations, the goal of any eating program is to "get the child to eat more food." Although increasing the number of foods the child eats is an important secondary goal, the main focus is to provide children and families with a positive mealtime environment and support them as they explore new foods.

Each girl with ASD who experiences problems with eating is unique and, therefore, requires an individualized plan to meet her needs. A comprehensive treatment plan includes a multilevel and multisensory approach that requires a commitment from parents and the professionals working with the resistant eater. For school-age children, it is important that the school team create opportunities to implement the plan during the school day.

Although each child is different, and the goals for the treatment plan must reflect the unique characteristics of the child, there are some general goals for all treatment plans. These include:

1. To create a safe, positive, and nurturing mealtime environment.

2. To expand the child's responsibility in preparing, consuming, and cleaning up at mealtimes.

3. To improve the child's oral-motor development.

4. To address all physical needs of the child during eating.

5. To provide multisensory exposure to new foods.

6. To respect the child's communication and response to eating.

7. To expand the child's repertoire of foods and create a balanced diet.

The plan is not intended to be adverse or punitive or to force or bribe the child to eat. Throughout, the focus is on exploration and learning about new foods and eating.

The written treatment plan will focus on three primary areas:

- Environmental controls
- Physical and oral-motor development
- Stages of sensory development for eating

The areas of the plan may be addressed individually, or all may be implemented simultaneously. Also, the plan should be written down and be easy to implement. The plan is not intended to include rigid and inflexible deadlines.

Environmental Controls

The first area to address in the treatment plan is environmental controls. There are a number of factors that should be addressed in the environment.

Guidelines and Strategies for Structuring the Environment

1. Design a consistent schedule that includes all meals and snacks. Post the schedule and use a timer to assist the child. Children who struggle with eating a balanced diet should only eat meals and snacks according to the schedule.

2. Select a setting with minimal distractions. In most cases, the kitchen table is the most appropriate setting for a meal. Some modifications may be necessary, depending on the child's age and size. Children should eat all meals and snacks at the designated setting.

3. Create a supportive climate with written, age-appropriate rules. A supportive environment respects the child and does not allow adults to invade the child's mouth without permission. Never discuss the child's eating habits or how much she eats during the meal. If the child exhibits inappropriate behavior during the meal, remove her from the table, letting her know that her behavior is sending a message that she is not hungry. The family should finish the meal. The child may receive a snack later according the schedule.

4. Select child-friendly foods and portion sizes. Select one menu for the entire family. A family meal should include a protein or meat, starch, fruit, and/or vegetable, and milk. Always provide the resistant eater with at least one serving size of a preferred food item. Consider using a smaller plate to encourage child-size servings. A smaller portion allows the child to see the results when taking a few small bites.

5. Address food jags. A food jag refers to the insistence on the same food, or the same utensils, or even the same setting, over long periods of time. Do not cater to the child's rigidity in wanting the same foods. Make slight changes in the presentation of the food or change the brand names. Provide the child with forced choices for food items and/or utensils. Be sure the changes are small and do not create anxiety for the child.

Environmental controls are the foundation for a solid treatment plan. In order for the child to learn about new foods, the mealtime environment must be positive and nurturing.

Physical and Oral-Motor Development

The second part of the treatment plan focuses on physical and oral-motor development (Ernsperger & Stegen-Hanson, 2004). Young girls with ASD may experience minimal to severe delays in oral-motor development, or they may not have received appropriate physical supports to promote successful participation at mealtimes. This part of the treatment plan, therefore, addresses the physical and oral-motor development necessary for eating.

Guidelines for Postural Control and Improved Oral-Motor Development

1. Improve awareness of posture and strengthen the muscles that assist in postural control. Include children in household chores that strengthen muscles. Sweeping the floor, washing the car, and carrying groceries are everyday chores that focus on posture and coordination.

2. Increase shoulder stability and trunk strength through a variety of age-appropriate activities, which include wheelbarrow walking and playing tug-of-war. Some children with decreased trunk stability benefit from added support such as a towel roll wedged on the sides of the body or behind the back when sitting.

3. Improve postural control, muscle tone, and general endurance necessary for eating. Be sure to use child-size chairs or booster seats with foot supports. The child's feet support the legs and help provide stability and balance her body needs for good oral-motor skills.

4. Improve oral-motor development. Many different methods are utilized in the treatment of oral-motor issues, and

---

it is suggested that parents work closely with occupational therapists and speech and language therapists to choose which one is most beneficial for their child. Some interventions use facial massage or stretching of the muscle fibers of the cheeks and lips, others incorporate the use of equipment such as whistles, straws, and so on, to improve oral-motor skills. Remember, it is up to the child to give permission for the adult to enter her mouth.

5. Increase muscle tone in the jaw, lips, tongue, and cheeks. Oral-motor activities designed to improve muscle tone can easily be implemented into the child's daily routine. For example, while the child brushes her teeth, she can work on building awareness of her mouth and explore moving her tongue from one side to the other. Or during the drive to school, she can sing silly songs that focus on facial actions.

6. Increase active movement of the tongue, lips, and cheeks to promote chewing. Children with oral-motor difficulties often resist foods that require extended chewing. Chewing is a partnership between the tongue, the jaw, and the cheeks. Therefore, offer a variety of chewing devices.

Sensory Development

The final part of a comprehensive treatment plan focuses on sensory development. Children learn to eat new foods through the developmental sensory stages of tolerance, touch, smell, taste, and eating. Toddlers often play with and experience foods while sitting in their high chair. As toddlers touch and smell new foods, they eventually begin to place small amounts in their mouths. These same developmental stages of learning about a new food can be applied to resistant eaters.

By Jana (age 27 with ASD)

My early 20s were quite challenging because I refused to touch any food. If as much as one piece of lettuce fell from my sandwich, I would declare the entire meal ruined. I survived on diet meal-replacement beverages during a six-month stretch and landed in the hospital weighing less than 95 pounds. My digestive system atrophied, and like a baby bird fallen from its nest, I had to be slowly nursed back to health. I gave up on meat after finding bits of bone and cartilage in a hamburger. The idea of chewing on decaying animal flesh makes me queasy. If I'm at a nice restaurant and another patron makes strange noises while eating, or chews his or her food in a particularly disgusting manner, I lose my appetite and literally stand up and leave.

My husband has accepted my strange and seemingly illogical eating habits. They can change on a daily basis. Because I dislike eating around strangers, we mostly order takeout and eat in bed while enjoying an episode of Star Trek *or Futurama. A couple of years ago, my husband introduced me to heart-attack-inducing junk food. Although I've enjoyed eating horribly and have an extra 25 pounds of fat jiggling about, I have begun shifting to a healthier lifestyle. Who knows what I'll eat in the future! Soylent green? Okay, as long as I don't have to touch it.*

Jana describes the experiences of a resistant eater and some of the long-term consequences. If a comprehensive treatment plan is not developed, eating challenges may continue into adulthood. Eating a limited variety of fruits, vegetables, and proteins can have a long-term effect on overall health. For example, one young woman reported only eating hot dogs for many years, which adversely impacted her health.

No matter the age of the individual, acquiring a taste for new foods may take several weeks or even months. Researchers have reported that it may take up to 10-15 exposures of a new food before a resistant eater is ready to move on to the next sensory stage of development (Shield & Mullen, 2002). Therefore, a comprehensive treatment plan should include multiple opportunities for exposure at each sensory level.

Guidelines for Creating Positive Exposure to New Foods

1. Select and implement daily activities for addressing each stage of sensory development: tolerance, touch, smell, taste, and eating. For example, begin the program by allowing a new food to be in the vicinity of the child. Tolerance begins with looking at a new food and allowing the food to be present at mealtime. It is important for the child to be reminded that she will not be forced to touch or eat the new food. After several days or weeks of focusing on tolerance, assist the child in exploring new foods through touch. Games like "Hot Potato" can be fun for the child and help to decrease anxiety over touching new foods. Be sure to include a variety of foods to pass around when playing food games.

2. Implement activities designed for learning about new foods either at the end of the meal or at a separate time dedicated to "Learning About New Foods." Identify on the meal/snack schedule a 10- to 15-minute planned opportunity for implementing the activities.

---

3. Have fun and avoid coercion. The goal of each lesson is for the child to lead the activities and enjoy learning about new foods. Strong and enthusiastic role models reduce the degree of food neophobia and the fear of tasting new foods, while assisting the child in learning about new foods. The use of a puppet as a role model is fun and beneficial, particularly for young children.

4. Use typical peers or siblings for support. In the home setting, invite one or two typical peers over to participate in the activities. For school settings, typical peers may be invited to play food games and be role models. Be sure to select children who will be supportive and compliant during the session.

5. Repeat the same sensory activity several times if necessary. Children learn through repetition and enjoy playing games they are familiar with. It may take up to 10-15 times of repeating an activity before the child is ready to move on to the next sensory stage.

6. Remember that children do not all like the same foods. Everybody has food preferences, likes, and dislikes. In order to be considered a "good eater," you don't have to like every food. A good eater is one who enjoys eating, likes a variety of foods from each food group, and can tolerate new foods. If a child truly does not like a food after 10 attempts at exposure, select another food from the same food group.

7. Provide your daughter many opportunities throughout the day to learn about new foods. Learning about new foods does not have to occur only at a mealtime. Be creative and provide a food-rich environment. This means that a child is exposed to plastic foods in the bathtub/shower, singing about foods in the car, and reading about foods at bedtime. A food-rich environment is one where the child feels safe to learn about new foods across settings.

Due to the nature of resistant eating and the individualized strengths and weaknesses of each child, it is important to start the journey into learning about new foods in a fun and exciting manner. First, it is essential for those working with resistant eaters to have adequate knowledge and skills for addressing eating issues. Seek out support and training. A collaborative approach within a multidisciplinary team will ensure the long-term success of the program.

Last, we cannot emphasize enough the importance of maintaining a well-balanced perspective when managing resistance with eating. Although extremely difficult at times, parents must bear in mind the long-term goals for the child and family while minimizing the focus on day-to-day struggles that each mealtime may bring. Mistakes may have been made in the past, but children are forgiving and will begin to move forward in their learning about new foods. Young girls with ASD have an innate ability to learn and experience new things at their own pace. We must respect their gains and celebrate their successes.

Conclusion

Whether you are concerned about sleeping, toileting, eating, or other behavioral concerns, there are some specific guidelines to follow. First, implement proactive strategies for addressing behaviors. Proactive strategies include examining the environment, teaching replacement skills, and utilizing reinforcement techniques. Develop appropriate schedules and routines that meet the needs of the child. Examining the purpose or the function of the behavior is an important first step for changing future outcomes.

After reading these stories and learning the strategies for addressing the challenges of behaviors, sleeping, toileting, and eating, we believe you will feel empowered to create change. You will now be able to appreciate and focus on your daughter's progress and accomplishments, because along with education and intervention comes knowledge and hope.

CHAPTER 3

Off to School

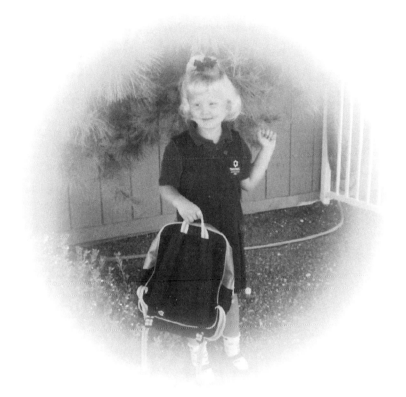

By Danielle (Mother of Mattie at age 6)

I had just dropped Mattie off on the playground with her kindergarten classmates and was walking to the car, when I realized I was still holding her lunchbox in my hand. Feeling totally exasperated after an already exhausting morning, I headed back toward the school, wondering how we even made it there in the first place. Our morning had begun with a major hair episode in which I'm not quite sure how we managed pigtails. Then, there was the memorable scene when Mattie's shoes weren't fitting right, because "I" failed to put her socks on the right way. I should have known that not putting on her socks "just so" would lead to a meltdown.

Not wanting to disturb Mattie on the playground, I decided to take her lunchbox to her classroom. Since the children were still outside playing, the classroom was empty when I arrived. I welcomed the quietness. As I walked by several rows of tiny tables and chairs, I glanced down at the neatly printed name tags on the table tops indicating the children's assigned seats.

Noticing that Mattie's name was not in the same place as two weeks prior when I attended her Halloween party, I began looking for her name tag. Then I saw what I had ultimately feared … an unmarked table in the back of the room facing the wall. As I walked over toward the table, a sick feeling washed over me, because deep down in my gut I knew that I had found Mattie's seat. Thoughts of my daughter's daily isolation from the rest of her classmates overwhelmed me. Unable to deal with my suspicions alone, I had hastily set out to find the principal. Seeing that I was extremely upset, the principal suggested we confront the teacher.

The walk to the playground seemed to take forever. I was so angry that my throat felt like it was closing up and I didn't know if I would be able to speak. However, I was determined not to let there be any discussion regarding this matter without my being present.

The teacher, who was totally taken off guard and obviously embarrassed, confirmed the inevitable. She told us that Mattie sat at the table in the back of the room because she had a hard time sitting next to the other children. Her voice shaking, she stated that she thought this was the best place for her. Barely able to keep my emotions under control as I thought how humiliating this setup must be for Mattie, I asked the teacher how anyone would even know Mattie was in the class when she didn't even have a name tag on the table that faced the wall! She couldn't make Mattie feel any more invisible if she tried. How could she treat any child this way? The next thing I knew, I blurted out, "My daughter is way too valuable to be wasted in your class!," and I walked away.

This heartbreaking experience made me realize that I would have to become my daughter's advocate, because her fair treatment could not be guaranteed by the type of school she attended or the qualifications of the teacher. I was not totally unprepared for this eventuality. I just hadn't expected that I would have to start in kindergarten.

Entering the world of public schools and special education can be a daunting, overwhelming, and sometimes exciting journey. Maneuvering the difficult legal vocabulary, intricate special education procedures, frequent lack of teacher training about students with ASD, and a plethora of professionals can make this a difficult experience.

In this chapter, we will review the elements of an individualized education program (IEP), including determining eligibility and least restrictive environment. We will also identify some of the most relevant related services to be provided to girls with ASD, including occupational therapy, speech and language services, and parent training. As girls with ASD get older, strategies for social skills training, bullying prevention, and transition to middle school will be explained. But first we will briefly review the special education laws.

The Education of All Handicapped Children Act, otherwise known as EHA or Public Law (P.L.) 94-142, was passed in 1975. This law mandated that special education and related services be made available to all eligible school-aged children and youth with disabilities. Since the time of EHA's enactment, federal funds have been granted to help state and local educational agencies provide special education and related services to children with disabilities ages 3-21.

In 1990, as part of its reauthorization by Congress, the EHA was renamed the Individuals with Disabilities Education Act, or IDEA (P.L. 101-476). The law was again amended in June 1997 as P.L. 105-17. In order for a girl with ASD to receive special education services within the federal guidelines of IDEA, the school and parents must conduct an assessment and find her eligible. We will review the eligibility process and how parents and professionals can work together to create an appropriate IEP.

School Daze

By Rosemarie (age 17 with ASD)

My memories of school were far from what would be considered normal. Many nights I lay crying in my bed, afraid that one of my school pencils might not be sharp enough. I was frustrated because I absolutely had to walk with my desk partner when switching classes and was not permitted walk alone. The slight cracks between the adjoining desks bugged me. Lunch time in itself was hell. I was afraid that I would miss recess or class afterwards. Therefore, I would pick two classmates every day and ask them "to sit beside me at lunch and play with me at recess." This was my typical day.

Girls with ASD may be identified during the 3- to 5-year-old period of development but most, like Rosemarie, are not identified until they enter school or much later (Attwood, 1999). As we discussed earlier, parents and professionals may not observe some of the early signs and symptoms because girls often display less intrusive or less aggressive behaviors than boys.

Whether your daughter is in preschool or has already begun kindergarten, if you have concerns about her development, contact the local school district for an evaluation for special education services. Parents may also choose to obtain an outside independent evaluation of their daughter to determine what services she might need.

In order for your daughter to receive special education services, the following steps must be taken by the multidisciplinary team, which includes the parents and school personnel:

1. Conduct an educational evaluation.
2. Determine special education eligibility.
3. Write an IEP.

Educational Evaluation

First, we will review the procedures for acquiring special education services through your local school district. All public schools receiving funding for special education services under the IDEA regulations must provide a free appropriate public education to children with disabilities. In order for your daughter to receive special education services to meet her needs and to help her learn the general education curriculum, the school must conduct a comprehensive evaluation to determine eligibility. Parents must give their informed consent before their child is evaluated. The evaluation is of no cost to the parent and must be conducted within a period determined by state regulations, often within 30-45 school days from the time the parents sign the consent form.

Once the parent has given an informed consent for the evaluation, a school multidisciplinary evaluation team will conduct the assessment. The team evaluates your daughter in a variety of areas, including social and emotional well-being, general intelligence, performance in school, and how well your daughter communicates with others. The role of the evaluation team is to get a picture of the whole child and her strengths and weaknesses as they relate to her education. The evaluation process may include a school psychologist, speech-language pathologist, occupational therapist, and other specialists who are qualified and knowledgeable about special education and autism spectrum disorders.

By law, parents are also important members of the evaluation team. Your specific concerns about your child's school experiences and developmental history are important in determining eligibility for special education.

Eligibility for Special Services

Once the evaluation team, including the parents, have completed their assessments and written their reports, the team will meet to review all the information gathered and decide if the child meets the criteria for special education and related services. For the child to receive services, the evaluation team must find her eligible within one of 13 categories identified under the IDEA regulations. Autism is one of those categories. Unfortunately, Asperger Syndrome is not one of the federal disability categories. Although many states have included Asperger Syndrome as part of the "autism" disability category, the federal regulations do not recognize Asperger Syndrome as a separate disability category. Therefore, some school districts are unclear about how to provide services for students with Asperger Syndrome.

According to the National Research Council (2001), students with "any autistic spectrum disorder (autistic disorder, Asperger's Disorder, atypical autism, PDD-NOS, childhood disintegrative disorder), regardless of level of severity or function, should be eligible for special education services within the category of autistic spectrum disorders, as opposed to other terminology," such as other health impaired or social emotionally maladjusted (p. 214).

Because the evaluation and eligibility requirements are extremely complex, parents must be knowledgeable of the specific requirements within the evaluation process and eligibility determination for special education services to ensure they receive services for their daughter. Parents may want to consider discussing these procedures with a special education advocate or an attorney in order to receive the appropriate services.

A Word of Caution

If the evaluation team determines that your daughter is not eligible for special education services, as a parent you have a right to receive information from the school about your procedural safeguards to challenge that decision. You may request an outside independent evaluation to be paid for by the school district.

Writing the IEP

The third step in the special education process is the writing of the IEP. If your daughter has been found eligible for special education and related services, the IEP team will meet to develop a written plan to address goals and objectives and specify the services your daughter will need to make reasonable educational progress. The IEP must contain information about the following areas:

- Present levels of achievement
- Annual goals and objectives
- Related services
- Participation with nondisabled peers
- Participation in district-wide assessments
- Transition goals for adolescence
- Measuring progress

Tips for the IEP Meeting

Attending the IEP meeting for the first time can be an overwhelming experience for parents. Danielle shares her reflections on the first meeting for her daughter with Asperger Syndrome.

By Danielle (Mother of Mattie, age 11)

I felt as though I was on trial as I walked through the school doors to attend my daughter's first IEP meeting. Upon entering the meeting room, the IEP team immediately greeted me and offered me a seat. The table was circular, but I felt like I was the only one on "my side." Was it just me, or was I the only person who got the chair brought in from the kindergarten classroom? The meeting had barely started, and I already felt like I was sinking.

The IEP team started the process by reciting Mattie's test scores, which I felt failed to reveal her true capabilities. How did they test her anyway? Was the test timed? Did they read the questions to her? Feeling very intimidated, I never asked these questions. I wondered if they even had an understanding of Asperger Syndrome.

Next on the agenda, the IEP team decided on Mattie's classroom placements, modifications, benchmarks, behavioral plan, and goals, all of which was totally overwhelming to me. As they each took turns helping me to understand my daughter's needs, socially, physically, and academically, I felt like I needed to share with them all of her good qualities.

After all, it's not easy to sit and listen to everything your child cannot do. Unfortunately, I was too emotional to find the right words.

After all was said and done, "I settled, signed my name; case closed."

Although not all initial IEP meetings are as focused on the student's weaknesses, parents must come prepared. The following illustrates some basic principles and describes what parents can expect.

1. The meeting should take place at a convenient time for both the parents and school personnel. It is important that parents attend this meeting; therefore, it may need to occur before work or during a lunch break.

2. Parents are encouraged to bring additional support to the IEP meeting, such as a person knowledgeable about their child who can act as an objective bystander, take notes, and help the parents stay organized with their agenda. This person can be a grandparent, an outside therapist, or a family friend.

3. According to the law, parents can prepare for the IEP meeting by making a list of their child's strengths and weaknesses. Create a draft of some of the learning goals to be addressed, but be open to compromise with school district personnel.

4. Parents are equal partners with school personnel in the development of the IEP. Therefore, all members of the team must communicate effectively and share what they know about the child's educational performance. Working as a collaborative team and writing a comprehensive IEP will ultimately affect the long-term outcomes for the child.

5. Parents do not have to sign the IEP document at the end of the meeting. If you need a chance to review the document and discuss it further, end the meeting and reconvene at a later date.

As stated above, the IEP addresses a variety of important areas for a successful educational program. For girls with ASD, there are some additional requirements to an IEP that should be considered by the team, including classroom placement options, appropriate related services, and curriculum modifications.

Placement Options

By law, educational placement decisions are based on the individual needs of the student and the identified services to be provided by the school. The placement should be in the least restrictive environment where the student has access to the general education curriculum and typically developing peer models.

Depending on the information gathered by the team, the appropriate placement may be in the general education classroom full time with supports and services. Indeed, most girls with ASD remain in the general education classroom with the appropriate supports, modifications, and services. Some girls may spend short periods of the day in a resource room with a licensed special education teacher. The resource room teacher can address social skills, study skills, and assist students in organizing and completing their homework.

By Nicole Charest (Teacher)

As I geared up for another school year, I began looking through my student portfolios in order to become familiar with my new learning family. This particular year, I had 20 students in my third-grade class: 8 boys and 12 girls. In reviewing each child's information, I came across the word "autism" as a diagnosis for one of my student's named Mattie. Being a fairly new teacher, I became immediately intrigued and challenged to have a child with autism in my classroom. However, I also knew that I needed to learn more about this disorder.

After reading some literature on autism, talking with my special education staff, and meeting Mattie and her mom, I began feeling more confident and ready for a successful year. In mid-August, I started planning my first few weeks of school – a crucial time of the year where I build my foundation for strong learning, respect, and risk-taking. In order to create a safe and nurturing environment, I knew that I needed to address Mattie's autism to the students. So, with the approval of Mattie's family, I created a plan. As a lover of reading, I decided to begin with a story titled Thank You, Mr. Falker *by Patricia Polacco. The main character in the story, Trisha, is dyslexic and has trouble learning. This powerful book demonstrates how the teacher and students worked together to help Trisha grow.*

By the end of the first week of school, I felt that the students had had enough time to get to know each other. That Friday afternoon I sent Mattie out of the room for some testing in order to speak to the other students about autism without caus-

ing her any discomfort. As I began by reading the story, I took time to stop and elicit the students' reactions to the character's feelings of inadequacy. I compared Trisha's character in the book to Mattie. Neither girl was weird, as the writer, Patricia Polacco, had so eloquently pointed out. Neither girl was sick or contagious. Their brains were just wired differently. In fact, I pointed out how we'd noticed that Mattie was a great reader, actress, and friend.

My next step was to define the word "autism." We discussed how Trisha saw letters backwards and upside down. I then explained that Mattie also experienced things a little differently from her peers. In an effort to help the students better understand autism, I set up a rotation center comprised of three different station: an auditory station, a tactile station, and a visual station. The stations were set up to allow the students to experience hands-on Mattie's perception of her surroundings.

- *Hearing: I played a radio really loud. This demonstrated how a normal voice may sound magnified in Mattie's ear.*

- *Touch: In a circle, we took turns poking each other in the arm. When it was my turn to get poked, I had the student pretend to punch me. This demonstrated how a poke or gentle touch could feel firmer or stronger to Mattie.*

- *Sight: In a circle, I had the children look at each other through the corners of their eyes. When it was my turn, I used a magnifying glass to look at the child next to me. I then blew up at that student saying that I didn't like his mean look and to stop looking at me. This demonstrated how Mattie's perception of someone's facial expressions could be misinterpreted.*

After we finished rotating through the stations, I explained that Mattie didn't always feel things this magnified; however, what may seem "average" to us often seemed more important to her. For example, Mattie was very concerned with the "Golden Rule" and was always trying to follow our expectations. I expressed that during these times, Mattie just needed some friendly help staying on the right path. I shared that just like Patricia Polacco's Trisha, who didn't like the other kids to baby her, neither did Mattie. I asked my students to treat Mattie as a friend and to be respectful of her needs and differences. We concluded by brainstorming ways we could help Mattie be successful.

When Mattie returned to the classroom later that day, I could see my students sitting up with pride that she was in our classroom. It was obvious that they cared about her. With the passage of time, I enjoyed watching a respect for Mattie cultivate and grow. By the end of the school year, she had achieved the "Golden Rule Award," and we all learned that autism was not such a scary word, but just one person at a time.

This teacher took the time to not only educate herself but the whole class about autism spectrum disorders. As a result, she set up a win-win situation for Mattie and her classmates. As parents and professionals, we all realize the positive impact a teacher like Ms. Charest has on our daughters' educational experiences.

What Else Does She Need to Succeed? Receiving Additional Services

Jazz (age 16 with ASD)

I didn't have any friends, and I was lonely. I couldn't help my autism; I didn't know how. I didn't even know I HAD autism at the time. I thought that what I was doing was perfectly natural. I guess it WAS natural, for autism. But what I was doing was the very reason why children made fun of me, and why people labeled me a "freak."

Then, my mom and I started doing things like having people teach me through Barbie dolls how I should act, putting small objects in my hand so I wouldn't do weird motions with them; and we also played Hooked on Phonics EVERY SINGLE DAY. If I didn't speak English, I wouldn't get what I want (which was usually sweets or toys).

She called it therapy.

Related services, or therapy as Jazz calls it, are defined as supportive services that are required to assist a child with a disability in benefiting from educational programming and receiving a free appropriate public education as guaranteed by law.

According to the National Dissemination Center for Children with Disabilities (NICHCY; www.nichcy.org), the purpose of related services are:

- to advance the child appropriately toward attaining the annual goals,
- to be involved and progress in the general curriculum (that is, the curriculum used by nondisabled students),

- to participate in extracurricular and other nonacademic activities, and

- to be educated and participate with other children with disabilities and nondisabled children.

If the multidisciplinary team determines the need for related services, they must first follow specific eligibility criteria, which may include further testing. A variety of related services are available if the student qualifies, including transportation, social work services, and physical therapy. The related services that are most often addressed and needed for children with ASD are occupational therapy, speech-language therapy, and parent counseling and training.

Occupational Therapy

Occupational therapy (OT) services can enhance a child's ability to function in the least restrictive environment (NICHCY; www. nichcy.org). In the following story, a family describes the need for OT starting when their daughter was very young.

By Tammy (Mother of Kate at age 2)

One weekend, my husband and I decided that it was time for our 2-year-old daughter, Kate, to appreciate the great outdoors by going camping with us. We had no other children, and we thought it would be an enjoyable experience for our little family.

Unfortunately, our first night did not quite go the way I had envisioned. We had a hard time getting to sleep, not because of the water splashing against the nearby rocks, but because of the sand that had found its way into Kate's sleeping bag, and her subsequent meltdown. She had always been very sensitive, almost startled at times, when someone would touch her. But now she was acting like there was sand paper ripping at her skin. After what seemed like an eternity, my husband and I managed to get every last grain of sand out of her bag.

As I lay awake listening to Kate's restless twitching and turning as she tried to fall asleep, I couldn't stop the many thoughts that kept revisiting my mind. "What am I doing wrong? Parenting can't be this hard. Everything with her seems like a major chore. Why can't she just be happy?" I finally was able to relax when I noticed Kate had drifted off to asleep.

The next morning after we finished breakfast, the three of us took a hike. Kate insisted on hiking in her Disney princess heals that mysteriously had ended up in her backpack. Well, you can only imagine how that turned out! While my husband continued the hike, Kate and I headed toward the community showers to freshen up. I had some anxiety on the walk to the showers thinking of how Kate felt about public restrooms. The unpredictable flushing sounds, the hand dryers, and even entering the stalls caused sensory overload for her. As we waited for our turn to use the showers, Kate seemed content to watch the other children enter and exit the shower stalls with their beach towels wrapped around them. Unfortunately, that peaceful moment was short-lived. I'm not quite sure if it was the pressure of the water pounding against her skin or the water temperature itself, but we will be remembered for years to come from the screaming and clawing that happened that day at Yosemite National Park – and it didn't come from any of the wild animals!

Kate and her family experienced first-hand some of the symptoms of sensory dysfunction and their impact on daily living. Kate is in need of OT for her over-sensitivity to sounds and textures.

Occupational therapy services in schools may include such services as:

- self-help skills or adaptive living (e.g., eating, dressing);
- functional mobility (e.g., moving safely through school);
- positioning (e.g., sitting appropriately in class);
- sensory-motor processing (e.g., using the senses and muscles);
- fine-motor (e.g., writing, cutting) and gross-motor performance (e.g., walking, athletic skills);
- life skills training/vocational skills; and
- psychosocial adaptation (NICHCY; www.nichcy.org).

Fine- and Gross-Motor Activities

Girls with ASD may require services from an OT to address fine- and gross-motor delays. According to the National Research Council (2001), children with ASD experience significant delays in motor skills as well as experience atypical sensory processing. The IEP team should discuss the need for therapy, and it should be written into the IEP as a related service. The OT may consult with the teacher and provide strategies for the classroom, and also work directly with the child in pre-teaching skills necessary for physical education. Some girls with ASD require a trained therapist to pre-teach the skills for playing dodge ball, four-square, and other typical childhood games. Taking the time to pre-teach these skills will ensure more success in gym class, on the playground, and at the park.

Fine- and gross-motor activities that may be implemented in the home and in the classroom include:

1. Obstacle courses
2. Bean-bag throw
3. Hopscotch
4. Jumping on a mini-trampoline
5. Wheel-barrow walking
6. Playing with squeeze toys
7. Popping bubble wrap
8. Finger-painting
9. Playing with play dough
10. Handwriting

It is important to schedule several opportunities throughout the child's day to provide fine- and gross-motor activities. Parents and professionals can join in and role-model appropriate play skills for the child. Keep the sessions short and playful. Add music to the fun to encourage participation.

By Danielle (Mother of Mattie at age 5)

A trip to McDonald's for lunch with my 75-year-old grandmother and my two small children should have been fun. However, I soon realized that this would not be the afternoon I had envisioned. First, my son, Nicholas, fell off the bench backwards onto the floor and screamed for 30 minutes. Then there was Mattie. Did I happen to mention, Mattie has sensory issues with clothes and at times doesn't want to be bothered with them?

After we ate lunch, Mattie and Nicholas joined the other children on the climbing equipment while I visited with my grandma. Our pleasant afternoon soon came to an abrupt end, when out of the corner of my eye I caught a glimpse of something that I hoped was not true. There was my 5-year-old daughter running around McDonald's totally naked! To my horror, she had also talked her brother into dispensing of his clothes. I was so embarrassed that I wanted to crawl under the table and never come out. Thank God I had Grandma there to help me quickly gather my children and escort them the restroom, while I squeezed myself up into the climber to retrieve those scratchy clothes that Mattie couldn't bear to wear any longer.

Just as I thought the afternoon couldn't have gotten any worse, I was proven wrong. On the way out of McDonald's, I was approached by a mother who thought it was her duty to tell me how awful I was as a parent. How could any mother allow her children to act that way in public? Already feeling frazzled and knowing that she didn't understand our situation, I said, "Go home tonight, kiss your children, and thank God that you are the perfect parent."

Sensory Processing Activities

Tactile defensiveness is just one area of sensory processing that can be difficult for girls with ASD. Mattie had difficulty with the texture of her clothing and felt calmer without clothes. Providing a variety of appropriate sensory experiences is another responsibility for the occupational therapist. Sensory processing disorders are common and should be addressed by a knowledgeable professional (Biel, 2005). A variety of assessment tools are available to identify the child's specific sensory needs, including (a) the *Sen-*

sory Profile (Dunn, 1999); (b) *Sensory Integration and Praxis Test* (Ayers, 1989); and (c) *Sensory Integration Inventory* (Reisman & Hanschu, 1992).

If you suspect your daughter is experiencing sensory dysfunction, here are a few activities that can be implemented in a variety of settings:

1. **Play with shaving cream in the bathtub or on a table.** This will help the child become desensitized to having different textures and smells on her hands. *Select a clean table and place a small amount of shaving cream on the top of the table. Have the child use her fingers to make a picture, create shapes, or bury small plastic figurines.*

2. **Swing from a rope.** This activity benefits movement, coordination, and the vestibular system. *Hang the swing outside or in the garage. Have the child swing for several minutes.*

3. **Dress up with different clothes and make-up.** This activity promotes an increased sensitivity to textures and focuses on fine-motor skills such as working with buttons, zippers, fastens, and ties. *Collect a variety of clothes with different textures and colors. Play dress-up and pretend play.*

4. **Play with musical instruments to assist with auditory sensitivities and vestibular (movement) input.** *Select a few hand-size instruments and play some music. Have the child move around the room while listening and playing music.*

5. **Use weighted blankets or vests at various times throughout the day.** This activity will help the sensory system and calm down a child who may experience hypersensitivities to texture. *Purchase weighted blankets or vests from specialty catalogs (see Appendix). Select 5-10 minutes per day to have the child wear the vest or lie with the blanket.*

As with the fine- and gross-motor activities, it is important to keep these activities brief, supervised, and scheduled throughout her day. Carol Kranowitz, author of the *Out-of-Sync Child* (1998), reminds us to follow the SAFE rules when using sensory motor activities:

SAFE Rules

S = Sensory-motor

A = Appropriate

F = Fun

E = Easy, economical, and environmentally friendly

Parents and school personnel can develop and implement short and fun sensory activities throughout the day in order to assist the child in managing her sensory system.

Speech-Language Therapy

By Rosemarie (age 17 with ASD)

Life is hard. And it is even more so for autistic people like me. I didn't have the capability to communicate clearly with my family. When I was 7, we went to visit my grandmother and then planned on a walk through a new mall. A beautiful carousel at the center of the mall attracted my horse-impassioned eye. On the carousel, I had the time of my life. I was determined to ride every pony. When my parents led me away before I had a chance to ride the last two ponies, I tried to tell them what I had missed, but all I could do was to scream. At the time, I thought they just didn't care. Unfortunately, my unintelligible screams were useless without a translator.

Communication skills are at the heart of the education experience. Schools are social environments that require students to be able to socially communicate with peers and teachers. Speech therapy is an ongoing related service for girls with ASD. Rosemarie could not find the words to appropriately express her need for riding the carousel and, therefore, reverted to screaming.

According to the American Speech-Language-Hearing Association (ASHA; www.asha.org), speech-language pathologists assist children who have communication disorders in various ways. They provide individual therapy to the child; consult with the child's teacher about the most effective ways to facilitate the child's communication in the class setting; and work closely with the family to develop goals and techniques for school and home.

Girls with ASD have a significant impairment of social communication skills, which include pragmatics, voice inflection, prosody, and nonverbal skills (Richard, 1997). A licensed and knowledgeable speech-language pathologist should utilize a comprehensive assessment that targets pragmatics.

Pragmatic skills include voice quality, intonation, eye gaze, facial expression and personal space. Girls with ASD usually have language but may need assistance with adapting or changing conversations or following the rules of conversations. Pragmatic language skills should be taught in a variety of natural settings utilizing different methods and peer role models. The IEP should reflect the following goals for addressing pragmatics (ASHA; www.asha.org):

1. Problem-solving skills
2. Staying on topic
3. Initiating a conversation
4. Changing topics appropriately
5. Ending a conversation
6. Requesting information and assistance
7. Giving information
8. Volume and pitch control
9. Personal space
10. Nonverbal communication skills

Nonverbal communication skills play an important role in our everyday social experiences. A quick wink of the eye, a thumbs-down, or folding of the arms can carry multiple meanings in a conversation. Individuals with ASD have deficits in the ability to demonstrate nonverbal communication skills and in appropriately analyzing the nonverbal communication behaviors of others. A speech-language therapist should include goals and objectives for teaching nonverbal communication skills in the child's program. Goals would include: using gestures, identifying facial gestures, appropriate eye contact, and body language, as identified in the following chart.

Examples of Body Language		
BODY PART	**ACTION**	**INTERPRETATION**
Head	Leaning to one side	Not understanding, listening, thinking
Face	Scowl (involves whole face: eyes are narrowed and squinted, nose is wrinkled, lips are pressed together, mouth is sometimes to one side)	Displeasure, intimidation, bullying, anger
Eyes	1. Wide open 2. Almost closed ("open just a slit") 3. Looking straight at someone or something (for longer than a glance)	1. Surprise, amazement 2. Disbelief, doubt 3. Staring (which is considered rude)
Eyebrows	Pulled close together (sometimes referred to as "knitted brows")	Thinking, confused
Mouth	1. Corners of the mouth lifted up (smile) 2. Corners of the mouth turned down 3. Opened wide	1. Greeting, happy 2. Sad, unhappy, disappointed 3. Surprise, shock
Chin	Lifted, pushed forward	Proud, tough, defiant
Body	1. Pointed finger 2. Hands on hips 3. Shrugging shoulders 4. Arms folded across chest	1. Giving directions, threat, getting in trouble 2. Frustrated, bored, questioning/expecting an answer 3. Questioning, don't know 4. Unapproachable, listening/taking in information

From *The Hidden Curriculum* by Myles, B. S., Trautman, M. L., & Schelvan, R. L., p. 7. Shawnee Mission, KS: Autism Asperger Publishing Co. 2004. Reprinted with permission.

By Charlotte (age 32 with ASD)

When you have ASD, it's like you have this totally different language that you have to learn to speak. If you don't know the language you don't "fit in" socially. I couldn't handle a large-scale social situation. Trying to conduct myself in a group of girls was extremely challenging. I had to follow along with the conversation in a language that I was unfamiliar with, being that it was high school and all the drama that goes along with girls. I personalized everything, which made it that much harder to get along with my peers. I remember being the outsider, always "looking in," watching other people enjoy life.

Young women like Charlotte are often isolated because of their inability to adapt to social-communication settings. Receiving speech and language services can assist with this deficit area. As required under the IDEA, a speech-language pathologist should be a part of the IEP team and work closely with school personnel in the area of pragmatics. Valerie's story below reminds us that as we teach communication skills, we must focus on generalizing the new skill in different environments and be flexible with the rules.

By Nina (Mother of Valerie, age 9)

My daughter, Valerie, always loved to tell other people the age of her grandmother. After witnessing this a few times, I sat her down and explained to her that it was not nice to tell other people's ages. I told her that if they wanted to tell someone their age, that it was up to them. She seemed to understand this unwritten social rule.

About a year later, we were in a restaurant. The servers were singing a birthday song to someone, and Valerie overheard a child tell everyone the age of the birthday person. Valerie immediately leaned over and whispered into my ear, "Doesn't that girl know that it's not nice to tell someone else's age."

As the child gets older, the role of the speech-pathologist may become more of a consultant. The social-communication needs of girls with ASD will continue throughout her school years. Speech-language therapy usually plays a vital role for girls with ASD throughout the school years and into adulthood.

Parent Training

An additional related service that may be written into the IEP is parent training. Parent counseling and training can help parents enhance the vital role they play in the lives of their children with disabilities. When necessary to help an eligible student with a disability benefit from the educational program, parent counseling and training may include:

- Assisting parents in understanding the special needs of their child;
- Providing parents with information about child development; and
- Helping parents to acquire the necessary skills that will allow them to support the implementation of their child's IEP (NICHCY; www.nichcy.org).

Gaining the skills that will enable them to help their children meet the goals and objectives on their IEP is a positive step for parents.

According to the Office of Special Programs (OSEP), parent training also assists in furthering the education of children with disabilities and will aid the school as it creates opportunities to build reinforcing relationships between each child's educational program and out-of-school learning (www.ed.gov/about/offices/list/osers/osep).

The IEP and Curriculum Modifications

Curriculum modifications may be necessary throughout your daughter's school years. Changes to the general education curriculum are determined and written into the IEP to maximize participation in the general education curriculum (Ebeling, Deschenes, & Sprague, 1994). A variety of modification may be utilized, including

- Increasing the amount of time for test taking
- Reducing the number of items on a test or assignment
- Reducing the amount of homework
- Preferential seating
- Use of visual aids
- Peer tutoring
- Use of technology such as computers and calculators

Determining appropriate adaptations and modifications is part of the IEP meeting. The IEP process can be an overwhelming experience particularly for parents who are new to the special education process. Take your time and do not hesitate to reconvene the IEP team if you have concerns over the amount and type of modifications addressed in the IEP. If you child's grades are failing and modifications are not being implemented, reconvene the IEP to make additional modifications.

Social Skills:
Oh Yeah, It's Not All About Me

By Jazz (age 16 with ASD)

My mom set some pretty amazing goals for me all those years ago. The evaluation team told her "at Jessica's current functioning level, it would be best to place her in a self-contained special education classroom. Mainstreaming may not be possible for her." So, basically, putting me in a class with regular kids wouldn't be a good idea because I rocked a little from side to side when I was nervous. I had a little tic with one hand, and that might disturb somebody else. What was so irritating to them was that nobody could predict when I would have a meltdown and bang my head on the floor. Never mind that I was what they call an "imitative" child.

My mother argued that putting me inside a classroom with kids that behaved in a regular fashion and having me imitate THEM was what was best for me. They didn't agree. So I went to a private school for a while until my mother could eliminate the behaviors that irritated them so badly and they felt that it was "safe" to put me into a class of regular children.

Jazz and her mom had difficulty explaining to the school the importance of including Jazz with her typical peers in order for her to learn important social skills. A qualitative impairment in social skills is a key characteristic of individuals with ASD. Social skill impairment includes an inability to form adaptive peer relationships, impaired symbolic and dramatic play, limited emotional expressions and nonverbal gestures, and a lack of joint attention and sharing experiences (NRC, 2001).

Who Teaches Social Skills?

Social skills training is an ongoing need for girls with ASD from early childhood through adulthood. Social skills acquisition occurs in all settings, including home, school, and community. In order for social skills training to be specifically delivered in the school setting, it must be written into the IEP. The IEP must emphasize the specific age-appropriate social skills to be addressed.

Who will teach social skills and how often? Anyone can teach social skills, including the general education teacher, resource room teacher, school counselor, social worker, school psychologist, speech-language therapist, occupational therapist, behavioral interventionist (a person with expertise in behavior analysis), paraprofessional, and peer buddies (selected peers who can assist the student in learning social skills).

No specific amount of time is required to teach social skills. They should be taught throughout the student's school day and in the most natural environment. The team should tailor social skills instruction to the unique needs of the student and deliver instruction in a variety of formats with multiple opportunities for practice. For example, the classroom teacher may choose to teach a few age-appropriate greetings utilizing a role-play format in the classroom. The teacher, perhaps with the help of peer buddies and other staff, must then assist the student in generalizing and practicing outside the classroom, to include recess, the cafeteria, field trips, and so on.

By Nina (Mother of Valerie, age 9)

One summer, 9-year-old Valerie attended a social skills day camp. After a few days of getting to know Valerie, the camp director spoke to her about her inability to limit her one-sided conversations. He asked Valerie if there was some cue that he could use to let her know when her stories needed to come to a close. Without hesitation, Valerie said, "Just tell me to wrap it up."

Social Skills Goals and Objectives

The goals and objectives for teaching social skills change over time. In the beginning stages, the focus is on play skills, sharing, and manners. Play is universal in early childhood and allows young children to explore their world and learn important social communication skills.

The following is a list of a few examples of short-term objectives that might be considered by the IEP team for young girls with ASD.

The student will:
- Initiate play on the playground
- Join a group to play
- Share toys and activities
- Follow the rules in a game
- Respond appropriately to losing a game
- Wait in line
- Ask for help from an adult
- Display appropriate manners in the cafeteria
- Respond appropriately to an adult saying "No"
- Initiate a greeting to a friend

This list is not intended to be exhaustive. For further social skills objectives for the IEP, refer to the Appendix.

By Danielle (Mother of Mattie, age 11)

As I walked through the double doors of Mattie's elementary school this afternoon and continued down the corridor toward her room, I paid little attention to the artwork and stories posted on the walls. When I reached her classroom and peeked inside, I noticed the teacher was still completing her lessons. Since the school bell was about to ring, I leaned back against the wall outside of the classroom and savored my last few minutes of peace for the day. As my eyes scanned the long wall of essays that the children had written about their "Best Friends," a piece of paper titled "TABATHA" and "written by Mattie" stared back at me. I moved in to take a closer look in order to make sure it was my Mattie who had written the story. It was!

As I read Mattie's story, tears welled up in my eyes. I felt honored that she had been chosen by the school principal to have her essay exhibited for all the school to see. More important, Mattie's written words allowed me to hear her voice in my mind and gave me a better understanding of what she was feeling. The word FRIENDSHIP took on a whole new meaning that day.

Tabatha

Written by Mattie – Fourth Grade

Tabatha is my best friend. She is in my fourth-grade class. She is helpful, thoughtful, and protective of me.

When it's time, we eat lunch together and then go outside to play. In class, if my teacher is explaining something that I don't get, I pass a note to my friend and she raises her hand and asks the teacher to let her help me.

She remembers to give me presents on my birthday, Christmas, and Easter. Tabatha is like my sister. I just love her. She is as lovely as a rose and sparkles like a diamond. I am lucky to have a friend like her.

She is as strong as anyone. Tabatha does not let any kids call me names or be hurtful. Tabatha thinks that she is my bodyguard.

It is wonderful to have her be my best friend. I hope that we can stay friends forever.

As our young girls become young adolescents, around 10-11 years of age, the social arena becomes more challenging with a stronger focus on friendship skills and conflict resolution. As a result, the goals and objectives for teaching social skills for adolescent girls become more complex with an emphasis on social communication, problem solving, and conversation skills. Mattie's story of Tabatha clearly expresses how important friendships can be for girls with ASD when they have acquired the appropriate friendship-making skills.

The following is a list of short-term objectives that might be considered by the IEP team for an adolescent girl with ASD.

The student will:

- Introduce herself to someone new
- Give someone a compliment
- Maintain an appropriate topic with peers
- Display appropriate nonverbal communication skills during a conversation
- Cooperate during group-work activities
- React appropriately to teasing or bullying
- Maintain appropriate physical contact with peers
- Explain and follow the rules for public versus private information
- Express empathy towards others
- Repair an interaction with a peer

A variety of social skills curricula are available to parents and professionals. For example, *Navigating the Social World* (McAfee, 2002) includes easy-to-implement lessons for teaching social skills. Other helpful sources include *Building Social Relationships: A Systematic Approach to Teaching Social Interaction Skills to Children and Adolescents with Autism Spectrum Disorders and Other Social Difficulties* (Bellini, 2006), *Super Skills: A Social Skills Group Program for Children with Asperger Syndrome, High-Functioning Autism and Related Challenges* (Coucouvanis, 2005), *S.O.S. – Social Skills in Our Schools* (Dunn, 2006), *and Social Skills Training for Children and Adolescents with Asperger Syndrome and Social-Communication Problems* (Baker, 2003).

Identifying Emotions

Hormonal changes start to occur during early adolescence, and estrogen begins to greatly impact the emotional stability of girls (Gurian, 2002). A young woman with ASD may begin to experience a wide range of emotional outbursts – from extreme anger to anxiety and depression. Mood disruptions, angry outbursts, and feelings of being overwhelmed by minor problems are typical during this developmental stage (refer to crisis management, p. 50).

The following is a list of some additional social-emotional goals to be considered during the IEP meeting.

The student will:
- Identify a variety of emotions
- Recognize signs of stress
- Utilize stress management tools
- Stay calm during stressful periods
- Seek out assistance from an adult when necessary
- Respond appropriately to conflict
- Apologize to peers when appropriate

Helpful sources for assisting children to identify emotions – their own and others' – include *Let's Talk Emotions: Helping Children with Social Cognitive Deficits, Including AS, HFA, and NVLD, Learn to Understand and Express Empathy and Emotions* (Cardon, 2004).

The emotional instability and moodiness of adolescent girls in general can be amplified for girls with ASD. "Autistic people tend to have strong feelings with little gradation, so the even minor problems can cause great stress," according to Zaks (2006, p. 234). Liane Holliday Willey (1999) goes on to explain that "[Anger] rips through Aspie teens. It has to. Too many things come at once to avoid a collision. I have had more than my fair share of angry episodes, so many I am embarrassed to recall them now" (p. 183).

Examples of extreme anger, anxiety, or depression should be reviewed with a medical doctor who has experience working with adolescents with ASD. Some of the symptoms of anxiety disorders and depression include excessive worrying, feelings of fear, extreme tension, poor decision-making, profound sadness, and dramatic changes in behavior.

By Rosemarie (age 17 with ASD)

School was hell wrapped in a hot winter fur. This one girl at school never wanted anything to do with me. All of my attempts to play with her resulted in rejection. One morning before class began, I decided to try a more daring approach. I barged in on her, anxious to be accepted into her friendship. When I ended up with the same negative response, I flung my hand deeply into her cheek, frustrated at the wound in my heart. As school progressed, my peers started to use my idiosyncrasies against me for their own fun.

A Word to Parents

Social skills training is not just for schools. Parents must play an active role in teaching and maintaining their child's social skills and daily living skills at home and in the community. Parents should focus on such skills as how to attend birthday parties, answer the phone, cross the street, and so on. Parents can provide multiple social opportunities outside of school for their daughters to practice newly learned skills. The following story shows Mattie's dad providing her with some real-life opportunities for practicing a new skill.

By Danielle (Mother of Mattie at age 8)

We try to use every opportunity we can to teach our daughter important life skills. My husband's choice of the appropriate time and place leaves little to be desired. His perfect teaching opportunity came one afternoon when he dropped my son and me off at the door of Target and said, "Take your time shopping. Mattie and I are going to work on a few skills." Although I did not quite understand what skills could possibly be taught in a Target parking lot, I proceeded into the store without further question.

My questions were answered upon returning to the parking area a while later. There was my sweet husband hiding under a tree at the edge of the parking lot watching our 8-year-old daughter cross the street. Back and forth she walked, watching only her feet. My husband kept shouting, "Eyes up, Mattie. Look both ways before you cross. The cars are not going to stop for you!!" I couldn't help but wonder what other people must have been thinking as he demonstrated just one more example of what extreme lengths we have to go through to teach our ASD children simple life skills.

Teaching Social Skills

Teaching social skills is a fundamental goal for girls with ASD from early childhood through adulthood. Several basic tenets apply when addressing social skills in school, in the home, and in the community (Sugai & Lewis, 1996).

1. **Select relevant and valued skills.** Not every social skill is relevant to the child, depending on her age. For example, very young children should focus on play skills and sharing, whereas older girls begin to focus on conversation skills, giving compliments, and fitting into the group. It is important that the skills are age-appropriate and meaningful to the student. As the student gets older, have her select the social skills she would like to address.

2. **Teach in a variety of settings.** Teach social skills in a variety of settings in order to encourage generalization. Social skills training must occur not only in the classroom but also on the playground, in the home, and in the community. The goal for any social skills program is generalization of new skills, which means the specific skill is selected and implemented by the child during the appropriate social setting. This is often a challenge for individuals on the autism spectrum. For example, generalization is difficult if the social skill is always taught in a separate setting, or if the student does not have several planned opportunities for utilizing the newly acquired skill.

Parents and professionals should be cognizant of the necessary steps to generalize social skills through a variety of instructional methods and in varied settings.

3. **Include positive peer models.** At school, peers can provide important examples to girls with ASD, and at home parents can ask siblings to model social skills. Selecting age-appropriate peers to model specific social skills can greatly enhance the learning experience (Marks et al., 1999).

In the following story, Eirianne, who is neurotypical, speaks of having a friend with ASD. She provides us with some valuable insight into how we can support such friendships in school and at home.

By Eirianne Kennelley (age 11, Mattie's friend)

My name is Eirianne and I am 11 years old. Mattie is my best friend. Life with Mattie has been amazing. I have learned that she is someone who looks at the world differently than I do, and that's okay. At my birthday parties, Mattie always wants to open my presents with me. On our play dates, she wants me to do her make-up, hair, and nails. We love to pretend that we are twins, and we always take our "American Girl" dolls wherever we go. We have been friends since we were born, and I hope to keep it that way. I have met many of her friends, and she has met many of mine. I have to say, Mattie has grown and seems much better at handling herself. I am very proud of her. At first, I noticed that she was different than my other friends, but as time went by, I was not afraid to show the world that I had a best friend with Asperger Syndrome.

Sometimes Mattie doesn't understand certain things, so I ex-plain them to her, but I feel I have helped Mattie through a lot of social situations by being patient. On my 10th birthday we had a Fear Factor Party. One of the games we played was eating candy gummy worms mixed into spaghetti. Mattie got very upset at first because she didn't know what to expect, but I promised her that I would do it with her and that it would be fine. When we look back at it, we laugh.

I love her like a sister, and I realized, no matter how different your best friend is from your other friends, they have the same thoughts, feelings, and as big of a heart as anyone else. Mattie just views the world differently, and sometimes she looks at it in a better way than you or I would. I am glad that I have Mattie in my life, or else I wouldn't be the person I am today. She is my sunshine that wakes me up every day. I know it isn't much to say about a friend I have known all of my life, but to me, just her face means a thousand words.

4. **Provide repetition every day.** Learning a new skill takes rep-etition. New social skills can be difficult to acquire; therefore, it is important to provide multiple opportunities for learning throughout the school day and at home. Generalization also requires planned opportunities for practice.

5. **Offer concrete feedback.** Every teaching lesson should in-clude concrete feedback. Concrete feedback should include both the positives and the areas needing improvement. Iden-tify one or two areas for the student to work on.

6. **Use a variety of instructional techniques.** Parents and pro-fessionals can utilize a variety of instructional methods for

teaching social and communication skills. This will encourage the skills to be generalized to the appropriate social situation. Instructional methods include:

- *Direct instruction:* Tell the student explicitly the rules for the social skill. Select a *teaching moment* (e.g., when both you and the child are comfortable and there are no interruptions and distractions) to directly explain and list for the child the appropriate social skill for the setting. For example, when attending a birthday party, directly teach the child how to give a gift.

- *Scripting:* Write or draw a social script for the student to review. As with our birthday example, write or draw the sequence of events for giving a gift at a party. Include specific verbal responses to gift giving.

- *Peer tutoring:* Select appropriate peers to practice new skills. Identify peers or siblings to assist with teaching a social skill. The peer can assist with role-playing the recipient of a birthday gift in the example above.

- *Scrapbook and picture albums:* Create a scrapbook of emotions or of pictures depicting different social acts. Many emotions can come up at a birthday party, and these should be taught prior to the event. Create a picture book of emotions that the child may observe during the party.

- *Social Stories™:* Developed by Carol Gray (1995), Social Stories describe specific social situations and provide an explicit response for the student. A Social Story explains why specific situations may arise and describes age-appropriate solutions. Social Stories include visual supports. Writing a Social Story for the birthday party is an effective tool for preparing the child for a new situation. Social Stories are short and can be read with the child repeatedly.

- *Role-play:* Select a specific social skill and have the child act out the correct responses. A role-play allows the child to practice new social skills and receive feedback from adults. The child can practice giving a birthday gift to a peer or an adult, for example.

- *Incidental teaching:* As opposed to formal, staged events, try to teach social skills in the most natural and inclusive setting. This is particularly important for ensuring generalization. Using the birthday party example, continue to provide feedback and instruction to the child when attending the party.

Using a variety of instructional methods will assist the student in learning the social skill through repetition.

By Danielle (Mother of Mattie, age 11)

Mattie's teacher pulled me aside the other day and said that she was concerned about Mattie passing notes in class. The teacher knew how hard we had been working on social skills and appropriate behavior in class, and thought we needed to teach Mattie how to discreetly pass notes instead of throwing them across the room. Of course, I was totally thrilled with the news, because this meant that Mattie was just doing what most typical fourth graders do. Oops, we forgot to teach her to how to be sly!!!

The Hidden Curriculum of Social Skills

The "hidden curriculum" is a set of unwritten rules or knowledge of how to react in social situations. They are skills that other girls just "pick up on" through observation or subtle cues that are crucial for them to fit in with their peers. As the above story demonstrates, Mattie was unaware of the hidden curriculum or the "subtle art" of passing notes.

Her teacher recognized that note passing was an important age-appropriate skill. However, in order for Mattie to be successful in this area, she would need to be taught how to pass notes using the following step-by-step instructions.
1. Check to make sure the teacher is not looking at you.
2. Use eye contact with the other student to signal the note is being passed.
3. Quickly pass the note under the desk.

Unwritten rules can be an extremely challenging concept for girls with ASD to learn; yet, they permeate all areas and phases of life. In order for our girls to be successful in developing these important skills, each rule needs to be broken down into steps and taught concretely. They will then need to practice these skills by role-playing in order to be able to eventually generalize it into the appropriate social situations. To learn more about the unstated rules in social situations, we recommend *The Hidden Curriculum* written by Myles, Trautman, and Schelvan (2004).

By Jana (age 27 with ASD)

I do not find bowling in a crowded house of lanes on a Friday night giggle-inducing. Amidst the perpetual chatter and my genetic inability to knock down more than one pin per evening, it's hard for me to find the fun factor. Don't get me wrong, I had a blast picking out gorgeous bowling shoes with contrast stitching and a custom-drilled ball, all of which fit perfectly into my matching bowling bag. To those around me, I look the part; that is, until I actually have to bowl. Have you ever seen a woman suffer a complete mental and emotional breakdown while bowling? If not, come watch me. I do for bowling what Happy Gilmore did for golf. Because I think I should be perfect at everything before I even try, it makes attempting new things more about suffering than satisfaction. One such evening, after my husband obligingly rolled the three games entirely by himself, I found myself strangely compelled to make him smile by lacing up my shoes and hitting the lane. It's true, even for an Aspie, love makes you do strange and unselfish things (even if flinging a heavy glittery ball down an oiled lane seems absolutely stupid).

There are some roadblocks to teaching social skills in a school setting, which include who will teach the skills, how long the instruction will last – in total or per session – where to teach the skills, how to assess for mastery, and so on. But Jana reminds us why it is important to continue to teach age-appropriate social skills. Young women with ASD will go on to create loving relationships and must learn the give-and-take within those social settings.

Mean Girls

By Charlotte (age 32 with ASD)

I attended my first all-girls' summer camp when I was 8 years old. I looked forward to the freedom of being away from my parents and doing pretty much what I wanted. Of course, I brought along all my favorite things from home (definitely an Asperger's thing) to keep me comfortable and busy. I still remember how excited I was on the first day of camp when I saw that I got the bunk in the corner. I could already visualize my posters being hung up on the back wall and my teddy bear propped up against my pillow. I was looking forward to an enjoyable eight weeks at camp.

I was assigned a "Big Sister" when I got there. All the younger campers had one; I guess for support. Although it was nice to have someone there for me, I didn't consider her my friend.

The camp had many traditions. Every Sunday night we would have a campfire ceremony. Each age group would sit in a line wearing our campfire hats (which looked like cowboy hats). Whoever had excelled at something that week got a feather to stick in their hat. Camp was pretty intense and very competitive, which at times made me feel like an outsider. It took three years to get my first feather, which was devastating.

I was made fun of and had to switch bunks from time to time, due to not getting along with the other girls. These girls would do mean things to me; I couldn't figure out why. I still remember this one girl who was in my bunk taking my deck of playing cards and throwing them up in the air and yelling "52 Pick-Up." She told me to pick them all up. And, I did it!!! These are the kind of things that set ASD girls apart socially. There was a place at camp called "silent rock," where we could go if we needed to think. It was a big rock near the bunk houses surrounded by trees. I found myself going there a lot.

Now, at the age of 32, I think back on these experiences and realize that it had to be something that I had done. It was my own behaviors that prevented me from getting along. Maybe it was my low tolerance for people, or the way I went into a defense mode in order to protect myself. I might have come across too harsh at times, which made me a target. All I know was that I couldn't stop. It was almost like having Tourette Syndrome. You just have this "THING," and you don't see it. Everyone else sees it, but you don't.

Charlotte describes her experiences with getting picked on and bullied as a young girl and not understanding how to react. According to McNamara and McNamara (1997), Mishna (2003), and Heinrichs (2003), children and adolescents with disabilities are considerably more at risk for being victims of bullying. Bullies target loners, and girls with ASD tend to be loners.

Based on the description of girls with ASD and the characteristics of individuals who are bullied, we can assume girls with ASD are at a higher risk for bullying encounters than their typically developing peers. Below are some of the characteristics of victims of bullying (Coloroso, 2003):

- Different in some way
- Disability status
- Cannot defend themselves
- Weak
- Alone
- Insecure
- Poor social skills
- Emotionally immature
- Appear weak and anxious
- Mental and emotional insecurities

These are some of the very characteristics that are often used to describe girls with ASD. We know that girls with ASD fit the stereotype for victims of bullying. And we know that bullying can lead to long-term emotional and mental effects (Heinrichs, 2003; Voors, 2000). Therefore, both parents and teachers must work diligently in preventing and ending all bullying towards girls with ASD. We will discuss the specific techniques for parents and school personnel to implement in order to create bully-free school environments.

What Is Bullying?

Bullying can take many forms – from physical aggression to mild teasing. Girls who bully other girls tend to be more passive and often less aggressive than boys (Besag, 2006; Crompton & Kessner, 2003; Heinrichs, 2003). Girls tend to intimidate, threaten, name call, and tease. That is, they give more verbal insults and are covert in their bullying attempts, such as "Your hair is lame," "You buy your clothes at Wal-Mart," "You are clueless and will never get a boyfriend."

Girls bully in different ways, which may be hard for adults to observe, including social intimidation, refusing to be friends, or gossiping. Girls bully through social exclusion: "We won't be your friend," "You can't play with us," and "There is no room for you."

Further, due to a lack of awareness and knowledge about autism and AS, teachers may unknowingly be bullying a girl with ASD in the classroom. For example, some teachers constantly demean students regarding some area of deficit, such as chronically telling a girl with ASD to "Pay attention," "Look at me," "Organize your books," "Write more clearly," "Stop daydreaming," "Turn in your homework," and "You are lazy." This type of negative attention is a form of bullying and must be taken seriously and reported to the administration. If girls are being harassed by their teachers, they should be instructed to talk to a trusted adult at school or at home. Parents should keep in close contact with school personnel to determine if their child is being harassed in the classroom.

What Are the Effects of Bullying?

Girls with ASD who are repeatedly bullied over long periods of time can become depressed and emotionally traumatized (Miller, 2003). It may be necessary to remind the school team and all adults that repeated teasing and name calling IS bullying. It is not acceptable for adults to say that a little kidding is O.K. or that everyone gets teased and that they just have to get over it.

According to the national organization Stop Bullying Me (www.
stopbullyingme.ab.ca), symptoms of victims of bullying include:

- Sleeplessness
- Moodiness
- Not wanting to go to school
- Withdrawal
- Acting out at home
- Depression

These signs should be taken very seriously. The stress and anxiety
of being victimized may be displayed in different ways by your
daughter. She may be more agitated at home and moody (Gurian,
2002). Girls with ASD may not understand that they are being
bullied or the extent of the bullying due to a language impairment and a general lack of understanding the social norms of a
group. Watch for signs and ask questions. Do not wait until your
daughter comes to you to talk about bullying. We can assume that
bullying is occurring, and therefore a plan must be developed, as
described in the following.

By Temple Grandin

From *Unwritten Rules of Social Relationships* (2005)

*If you fit in, life is easy. If you don't, that's when all the teas-
ing and bullying starts. For kids on the spectrum, it can be
pure hell. (p. 20)*

Important

When adult awareness and supervision increases, bullying decreases.

Steps to Prevent and Stop Bullying

The school is responsible for creating a safe and predictable learning environment. Bullies will wait until no adults are around. Lunchroom, hallways, school bus, locker rooms, bathrooms, and before and after school are favorite places – these are the areas that must be addressed by the entire team to ensure that girls and young women with ASD are not alone and vulnerable. Adult supervision and activism against all types of bullying is its greatest threat.

Parents and professionals can work together to create a safe learning environment by following these specific steps (Gray, 2004; Twachtman-Cullen, 2002):

- Educate all staff and adults on bullying prevention and signs of bullying
- Teach all girls with ASD how to react to bullying attempts
- Take immediate action against the bully. The quicker the intervention occurs, the more likely the bully is to cease the behavior
- Make it a school-wide program
- Recognize small acts of bullying
- Increase the student's social network by identifying an accepting social group

- Identify a safe person or place within the school where the child can retreat for safety
- Role-play and practice assertive responses to teasing (e.g. "So What!")

When teaching a girl with ASD how to react to bullying, it is important to role-play a variety of bullying situations (Gray, 2004). You may consider videotaping the role-play session and using the videotape as a teaching tool. The videotape would include the child appropriately responding to a bullying attempt that is role-played with a peer. The videotape allows for greater repetition through watching the tape and reviewing the correct procedures for stopping a bully. Review the various methods for teaching social skills and utilize them to teach how to react to bullying. These strategies should be ongoing and addressed in an age-appropriate manner.

If as a parent you have attempted to speak with school personnel about bullying encounters in your daughter's school, and if the school is reluctant to acknowledge the bullying or to make any changes, it may be necessary to reconvene the IEP team and add requirements to address bullying prevention. There are several areas in the IEP where the multidisciplinary team, including the parents, can address bullying prevention objectives.

1. **The Behavior Intervention Plan (BIP).** The BIP is written to proactively address areas of weakness in the student's behavior. One purpose is to develop objectives and teach proactive social skills. The BIP is, therefore, written to include objectives for the student to learn the social skills to prevent bullying from occurring and how to react to a bullying attempt.

2. **Supplementary Aids and Services.** This section of the IEP is written to address the need for services provided to the student to ensure success in the general education environments, which include non-academic settings and activities, such as recess, lunch, before and after school, and athletic activities. The team may determine and write in this section that the student is to be supervised at all times, which may include a peer buddy. The team may also determine that further teacher training in bullying prevention is needed in order for the student to be successful.

Take detailed notes of all phone calls or meetings you have with school personnel. Write down in a special notebook the specific topics discussed and the date of the communication. Well-written documentation may be needed if further steps are to be taken to stop bullying in schools.

Parents can also continue to take steps outside of school to support their daughter in her growth and maturity by doing the following (McNamara & McNamara, 1997):
- Develop your daughter's strengths outside of school (e.g., art)
- Have your daughter join a group with the same interests
- Focus on her talents
- Practice and teach your daughter ways to interact with others during group outings and special events
- Continue to teach age-appropriate social skills at home

Just a Thought

Ask the PTA for a few dollars to buy signs saying "Bully-Free Zone." Place signs around the school to promote a safe a healthy environment and follow up!

By Sherry (Mother of Amanda at age 7)

It would be another attempt of trying to find something for Amanda to do after a difficult first year in school. There are limited activities for young children to learn one on one, but as her mother I knew that finding her gifts was the only way to keep her focused.

After noticing that Amanda had drawn her own set of pictures for her ABCs, instead of cutting out the pictures that were given in her kindergarten class, I thought art might interest her. I contacted the president of our local art association, Mrs. Lillian Foulks, and asked if she knew anyone who taught art to young children. She knew of some classes; however, they were not one on one and she wasn't certain what age student they were aimed at. My heart sank because I knew that this would not work for Amanda.

As the conversation continued, feeling at ease with her gentle voice, I asked Mrs. Foulks if she would be willing to teach her. There was a short silence on the other end, followed up by, I'm 70 years old and have never taught a 7-year-old one on one, but I guess I could try." Mrs. Foulks then gave me the list of supplies to bring and ended, "The lesson will be two hours long and it will be on a trial basis." My heart sank again, knowing that Amanda would not make it for two hours at a strange woman's house, but I decided to check Mrs. Foulks's references anyway.

Amanda was thrilled at the idea of art lessons. She could hardly wait to have her very own canvas, brushes, and paints. Tomorrow could not come soon enough for her. When we arrived at Mrs. Foulks's house, there stood a white-haired, beautiful lady with a sweet smile. I almost felt guilty that I had not told her about Amanda having a hard time sitting still, but I didn't want to jeopardize this opportunity. I left her with my cell phone number, in case she needed me. I then drove around the corner and parked, waiting for the phone to ring. I checked my phone a few times wondering if the battery was dead, but there was no call.

After two long hours of anxiety and anticipation, I drove back around the corner, parked, and went to the door. They came to the door dripping with paint with huge smiles stretched across their faces. Amanda was radiant in a way that I had never seen before. "Hi, Mommy," she said grabbing my hand, leading me in to see her painting. "This girl can paint!" replied her teacher. My heart jumped for joy at the compliment. My eyes were drawn towards this beautiful painting of watermelons that Amanda created. In my eyes, Amanda looked more beautiful than ever. Somehow, she suddenly looked so different to me. Who was this little girl?

Every week there was a new painting more beautiful than the last, sunflowers, tulips, and daisies. Our lives began to change. No longer was Amanda this pretty little girl that couldn't keep still, she was an artist. The road ahead would become a little easier. The difference would be perspective. Looking through different eyes, there was a picture of hope.

Bullying in schools is an increasing concern. Girls with ASD are easy targets, and, therefore, require a systematic plan for decreasing bullying opportunities and for responding appropriately. Sherry began to focus on Amanda's talents and strengths. By advocating for her daughter, she helped to build her self-esteem and self-confidence, which is ultimately the best tool against bullying. Parents and professionals should take an active role in protecting our girls from bullies and creating a positive self-image.

Sibling Relationships

By Karen (Mother of Rosemarie, age 17)

I was bursting with pride and enthusiasm the day we took our son Matthew to college. It was an emotional experience for our family. He was our first child, and he was moving eight hours away from home. To help kick off our son's new venture, I insisted the entire family travel to Notre Dame. At the time, our 9-year-old, autistic daughter, Rosemarie, was having seizures and not doing well; however, I was determined that we all share in the moment.

When we arrived at the beautiful campus, we were soon surrounded by all the other proud, smiling parents who were savoring the last moments with their children before releasing them into their new surroundings. I, on the other hand, was thinking of how hot and miserable Rosemarie looked and wondering when she was going to have the big meltdown.

After about 10 minutes of walking around the campus in the heat, the inevitable happened. Rosemarie began cursing loudly about our choice of hotel. Our hotel was very nice, but it was not the same hotel we had stayed at during our previous visit to the campus. The stares from other people began, and we knew we had to leave fast. My husband drove Rosemarie and me back to the hotel, while leaving our two boys behind to check in. He then returned to the campus to get Matthew settled in. Our planned three-day college adventure ended that same day. On our way home that evening, we stopped by our son's dorm room. I got out of the car to say a quick goodbye, and I cried all the way home.

At times, having to expend a tremendous amount of energy on Rosemarie at the expense of her siblings is painful. I have become an avid "people watcher." I am always aware of other families sharing their lives in ways in which we are unable – such as being able to share uninterrupted moments with my son.

Our definition of the nuclear, traditional family has changed over the past 50 years. Girls with ASD may live in a home that includes stepfamilies, half-siblings, grandparents, and single-parent homes. Families who have a daughter with ASD may also have other children with special needs. Given these variables, the sibling relationship takes on a new meaning. As we can see from the example above, there can be a great deal of tension and stress when dealing with siblings and girls with ASD. Having a sibling with a disability can create family issues, including:

- Resentment for spending too much time and paying extra attention to the girl with ASD
- Lack of understanding about the needs of the sibling with a disability
- Anger when the sibling with a disability "gets away" with exhibiting inappropriate behaviors
- Miscommunication between siblings during social settings (Harris & Glasberg, 2001).

All of these areas can lead to stressful family situations. Families who have girls with ASD often experience higher rates of stress and demands. Parents of daughters with ASD have a fast-paced life with therapy appointments, school meetings, and doctor's visits. A fast-paced hectic lifestyle is not conducive to creating a safe, secure, and balanced household. Therefore, time and attention are commodities.

When family time is at a minimum, it can be difficult to provide equal quality time for all the children in a household. Competition for the parent's attention can lead to feelings of guilt and resentment (Feiges & Weiss, 2004; Hart, 2001; McHugh, 1999). It may also lead to the typical sibling treating the sister with ASD as a burden or an embarrassment. Keep in mind that sibling competition occurs within all families at varying levels. Acknowledging that sibling rivalry and competition is a normal part of growing up in a family can help to reduce the guilt.

According to Donald Meyer (2004), director of the Sibling Support Project (www.thearc.org/siblingsupport), "Typically developing children should be allowed to experience a normal sibling relationship where sometimes they may tease or misbehave." Sometimes the sibling may tease his or her sister with ASD.

Do not automatically take the side of the child with special needs. It should not always be the typically developing siblings who have to make amends and change their behavior. Open communication and family meetings will help to resolve these issues of competition and resentment.

As part of the family dynamics, the typically developing child may also resent that the sister with ASD is allowed to circumvent the family rules or "get away" with more inappropriate behavior. The rules should be the same for all. If the typically developing sibling is complaining that things are not "fair," listen to the complaints. Never tell your child that it is "O.K." for one sibling to break the rules because she has a disability. Acknowledge the sibling's feelings, "It sounds like you are pretty upset because Jennifer did not get punished for breaking the Play Station." Allow the child to voice his concerns and take them seriously.

In the following story, Luke shares his initial resentment of his sister and the frustration he felt by her outbursts. As an adult, he can now understand her idiosyncrasies and use it as a bonding experience.

By Luke (Brother of Rosemarie)

Growing up with Rosemarie has never been easy. She has always demanded all the attention from our parents. It would be easy at times to be thinking "she is so spoiled," but we knew that she couldn't help acting the way she did, so my brother and I never really resented her. When we were young and in school, she would draw on our homework, shut down the computer while we were on it, and sometimes keep us awake at night with her talking and rocking. It is frustrating when nothing works to stop the behaviors. Her limitations limited us.

She is almost 18 years old now but still acts like a little kid. The thing about little kids is that there is never a dull moment when they are around. Over the years we would playfully tease or trick her into doing things that a typical person her age would never do. Once she realized she had been "had," she would mimic our behavior and try tricking us into something that is so obvious. Her child-like playfulness and gullibility has allowed us to both bond and share many laughs together.

Be aware of signs of trouble ahead concerning sibling rivalry. As the parents, you must be good detectives in managing and observing meltdowns, tantrums, and aggressive behaviors. If your typically developing child seems agitated, anxious, and angry, there may be some underlying issues and concerns that need to be addressed. Acting-out behavior and aggression are often symptoms of sadness and resentment (Meyer, 2004). Look at the situation through the eyes of the typically developing sibling. What is the underlying cause of the aggression: jealousy, lack of parental attention or possibly too many responsibilities around the household? As the adult, you must be consistent and set high expectations; there should be no tolerance for physical aggression by any of the children in a household.

"Catch 'em Being Good"

Use positive reinforcement and specific praise when the typically developing sibling is demonstrating appropriate behaviors. Set your goal at 10-12 specific opportunities during the day when you will give praise to the child for staying calm and being friendly.

Creating a safe, happy, and nurturing family environment is a universal goal for all parents. Here are a few guidelines to help you meet your goal (Harris & Glasberg, 2003; Hart, 2001; McHugh, 1999; Meyer, 2004; Sakai, 2005):

1. **Remember that typically developing siblings may over-compensate and overachieve.** Often siblings feel they cannot be themselves or have to prove themselves to be better than others. This can lead to resentment. The typical siblings may appear to be maintaining their behavior and doing well in school, but there may be some underlying concerns to be discussed. Take time each week to listen to their concerns and watch for any signs of problems.

2. **Teach specific age-appropriate information about ASD to typical siblings.** Provide them with the facts and rehearse with them how to share information with their peers. Teach specific behaviors for dealing with peers who may bully or tease. Be sure to practice how to respond to teasing so that your child is feeling self-assured in his or her skills. According to Harris and Glasberg (2003), even though siblings are accustomed to the word "autism" and seem comfortable with the term, they continue to need education throughout their development. It is also important to carefully explain some of the misconceptions people may have about ASD.

3. **As siblings get older, make sure they are part of the family plan when discussing long-term plans for their sister with ASD.** Meyer (2004) suggests that siblings be given a choice when deciding matters about their involvement with the future of their sibling with a disability. Thus, parents and educators should include siblings when discussing transition plans and future living arrangements. Although most girls with high-functioning autism and AS will lead independent lives, they may always need family support and guidance. This should be discussed openly.

4. **Remember that brothers and sisters have a right to their own lives, separate from their sister with ASD.** Give each child undivided attention, even for short periods of time. Plan some time throughout the week to do a one-on-one activity with each child. Provide typical siblings opportunities to excel in their own activities. This will foster self-worth. While it is often difficult to fit another activity into a busy schedule of appointments and school, it is vitally important to address your children's individual needs. Take time to talk about topics other than ASD.

5. **Do not put brothers and sisters in the position of caregivers with adult responsibilities** (Harris & Glasberg, 2001). The typically developing siblings should not be held responsible for the safe keeping of their sister. They should be allowed to be just siblings. Nevertheless, parents should teach typically developing siblings how to best handle their sister in different situations, such as appropriate ways to interact and play. Often it is difficult for the typically developing sibling to connect with a sister with ASD. If play skills are delayed or if stereotypical behaviors interfere with play, there may not be many opportunities for positive play. Look for opportunities for a simple game of catching a ball, popping bubbles, or jumping on a trampoline together. This time should be highly supervised so that both siblings experience a positive outcome.

By Matthew (Brother of Rosemarie)

The hardest thing for me is to see Rosemarie when she is frustrated. You feel so helpless when she is out of control. I remember the Christmas when she was in second grade and blurted out in class, "I have a secret that will ruin everyone's Christmas!" The teacher rushed her out the door into the hallway before Rosemarie could reveal the secret that Santa Claus wasn't real.

Rosemarie says the most incredible things. Her intelligence, wit, and insight are gifts that add richness to our lives and compensate for the hard times. I wonder if she would be so amazing without autism?

6. **Have high expectations for all the children in your household.** The rules should be the same for all. Matthew shares his concerns about his sister's out-of-control behavior. Siblings need assistance when confronted with these kinds of behavioral issues. It is important to teach the typically developing sibling how to handle tantrums and meltdowns. Create a family plan for how to deal with meltdowns when out in the community. As parents, we all make mistakes along the journey. Remember that children are forgiving. If, during a crisis, you blamed the typical sibling for the problem, take some time after things calm down to explain your mistakes. Talk about preparing for a crisis together.

By Myron and Danielle (Parents of Mattie)

There are many times when my husband and I feel that both of our children are affected by autism. We're not quite sure who gets the shorter end of the stick – Mattie, diagnosed with Asperger Syndrome at 5 years old, or our typical son, Nicholas. Because most things seemed to be a challenge for our daughter, it is not uncommon for us to constantly praise her accomplishments. Although we are extremely proud of our son, we have always just expected him to do well. Because we are so wrapped up in "her autism," he just has to be good.

We take great pride in both of our children's individual sets of gifts. Mattie works so hard at things we just take for granted and takes such joy in things we sometimes overlook that she is a constant reminder of what is precious in life. Nick is admirably loyal and accepting towards his family, and seems to find the positive in everything and everyone. With their strength and constant willingness to go the extra mile, it is truly a privilege to be their parents.

Having a sibling with a disability can be a rewarding and growing experience for the entire family. The Wendel family has focused on the individual strengths of each child. Having a sister with ASD can promote emotional maturity and understanding in Nicholas that he might not otherwise have demonstrated.

Adult siblings often report a great sense of self-assurance and capacity for empathy and understanding of others. Important virtues are developed by having a sister with ASD, which includes patience, tolerance, empathy, and compassion. As Mattie's brother Nicholas has said: *"When someone makes fun of my sister, it may not feel like a broken bone, but it still hurts."*

Middle School: A World of Its Own

By Elizabeth (age 13 with ASD)

My teachers started talking about transitioning to middle school in October. They said we needed to be organized and responsible. These words started to make me very nervous, because no one had ever told me that I was not responsible and organized. How do you become responsible and organized? I asked my mother many times throughout the year if I was a responsible and organized person. She would tell me that I was working on it and that it takes time, so not to worry.

The first day of middle school was very scary. I thought I would end up in detention all the time for getting lost and not being responsible. However, my teacher had posted a copy of the schedule on both sides of the hallway as well a large list of seventh-grade names that told you what room to go to for first period. There was also a teacher assistant who would check on me in the hallways to see if I needed help with my locker. Since Mom bought me a combination lock over the summer to practice on, I was able to open my locker in 7 seconds. Middle school wasn't as scary as I thought it would be. In fifth period I had a social skills class, and the teacher said she would help us get our notebooks organized. She gave out pocket dividers to put our work in so it wouldn't get lost.

I just love being in middle school. I'm working on being a responsible student, but I still need a lot of help keeping my notebook organized. My mom tells me to take it one day at a time and to ask for help before I get frustrated. Her advice is usually good since she has worked in middle schools for many years.

The thought of sending your beautiful, innocent young daughter into the scary halls of middle school can be overwhelming for parents. The changes from elementary school to middle school seem monumental, including passing periods, multiple teachers, hallways, lockers, and changing into P.E. clothes. Luckily for Elizabeth, her parents and teachers assisted her in making the transition.

For young women with ASD, the transition to middle school must be approached in a systematic and well-planned manner. We will examine three phases of middle school transition planning: before the student arrives, the beginning of the school year, and ongoing assessment of the transition plan.

Before the New School Year

The first phase in middle school transition planning begins in the spring prior to entrance to middle school. This is the time to begin working with the middle school team in planning for a successful transition. The steps in this transition phase include the following – on the part of both schools and families.

- **Provide training.** Many teachers are unfamiliar with high-functioning autism and Asperger Syndrome and need additional training (Frohoff, 2004). Most school districts or state regional education centers have autism consultants available to provide training to classroom teachers. The training should include all staff members who will come in contact with the student, including cafeteria staff, custodians, and bus drivers.

- **Review current IEP and BIP.** The IEP from the elementary school may not be adequate for the rigors of middle school. The multidisciplinary team, including the parents, should review the IEP. Make sure the BIP addresses the issue of bullying. Bullying tends to build in the later elementary school years and peak in middle school (Rousso & Wehmeyer, 2002). Unfortunately, most teachers see this as a passing phase and do little to prevent bullying from occurring. Middle school students have very little tolerance for differences. Therefore, the IEP and BIP must identify the procedures for preventing bullying.

- **Select courses and teachers.** The school team, including the parents and the student, should take time to review the available courses. Select courses and teachers based on the student's strengths and needs. An additional consideration is the teacher's strengths and weaknesses in working with students with special needs (Frohoff, 2004).

- **Visit the school.** It is not too early to visit the school and practice moving around the campus. According to Elizabeth's mom, who is a special education teacher and a parent, the team arranged for a school visit for Elizabeth in the spring.

By Karin (Mother of Elizabeth, age 13)

As a middle school special education teacher and a parent of a daughter with ASD, I have had some positive experiences with transitioning students to middle school. First, our school counselors start the process by visiting the elementary schools and discussing classes and schedules with the incoming students. Our school invites all of the sixth-grade classes from the incoming schools to take a tour of the school and have lunch with the seventh-grade students. Then in May our school has a sixth-grade orientation for students and parents in the evening. They watch a short movie the students made. It shows a day in the life of a seventh grader starting from the bus in the morning to after-school activities. It also has tips and myths from students about their first days and months of school. There are a few lockers set up for the students to practice using a combination lock. (We supply other kinds of locks if combination locks are difficult for some students, and we give our students end/corner lockers so they only have one person beside them. They don't share lockers either.)

We also provide one-on-one tours for students who need extra assistance. I take them around the school and introduce them to our hall monitors and security guards. They get to spend an hour in a core class, eat lunch in the cafeteria, and then spend an hour in an elective class. We also spend some time in the hallway, especially during passing periods, and discuss the noise level, crowds, and getting to class on time. If students need an individual tour after this, I will arrange for a teacher assistant to walk them through a typical day. We usually use an assistant they are familiar with from their school.

- **Review homework policies and modifications.** Middle school teachers usually share a strong belief in assigning homework, which can create anxiety and problems for students with ASD (Myles & Adreon, 2001). Homework can become a difficult part of middle school if it is not adequately addressed prior to the start of the school year. The multidisciplinary team, including the parents, should discuss any modifications to homework as part of the IEP meeting and write specific modifications into the IEP. Simple modifications to homework may include allowing more time, using a calculator, using a computer, reducing the amount of homework, and providing peer tutors.

Start of the School Year

The second phase of the transition planning begins as the school year starts. This is the period for the school team, the parents, and the young women with ASD to identify areas of concern and create a proactive plan.

- **Identify before- and after-school zones.** Middle school students tend to "hang out" with their friends before and after school. Hanging out is not always easy for young women with ASD. Therefore, school personnel and parents should develop a plan for where and with whom the student will be hanging out. Remember, bullies target students who are alone, so the plan should ensure a safe environment (Wagner, 2002).

- **Practice going to classes and locker.** Middle schools only allow a few minutes for passing between classes. It is important that someone is assisting the young woman with ASD in managing her time and getting to class. A positive peer buddy can be helpful with lockers and managing hallways.

- **Review lunch time procedures.** The cafeteria can be a chaotic and stressful environment for young women with ASD. Students are expected to move independently through the lunchroom and socialize with peers. It is important to identify an appropriate social group for the young woman to sit with and practice the routine of the cafeteria. It may also be necessary to examine the student's sensory needs and how they may be affected in the cafeteria.

- **Select a safety zone and staff.** There may be situations when a young woman with ASD will feel overwhelmed with the school environment and needs to speak with a trusted individual in a safe place. The team should identify who will be available in these situations and how the student can attain access to the safety zone. For example, the student may be directed to go to the counselor's office if there is a crisis in class or if she is being bullied.

- **Assist with organizing schoolwork.** Color coding each subject can aid the student with organizing assignments: Math is blue, English is red, and so on. It may also be helpful to have a peer buddy check school folders and assignment notebooks for accuracy. The peer buddy is a highly dependable, trustworthy student who can assist the girl with ASD in the classroom.

Ongoing Assessment of the Transition Plan

The final phase of transitioning to middle school is ongoing assessment of the transition plan and its overall efficacy. The school team, including the parents and the young woman with ASD, should plan on reconvening after the first few weeks of school to ensure the plan is appropriate and is meeting the needs of both the staff and the student. The team should consider the following:

- **Need for ongoing staff development.** Educators, including paraprofessionals, require ongoing support and training in working with students with ASD. Autism specialists and consultants should conduct a needs assessment to determine areas of weakness and plan for future training, as necessary.

- **Review of discipline referrals and grades.** It is important to check on grades and any discipline referrals early in the school year (Frohoff, 2004). The team can determine if further modifications need to be written into the student's IEP or if the BIP needs to be updated.

- **Overall success of the transition plan.** In order to be proactive, the team should regularly assess if the student is being successful and is adjusting to the new middle school environment. The team should ask parents about any issues arising at home. Also, it is important to directly ask the student how she feels the school year is going and if she is feeling successful.

By Karin (Mother of Elizabeth, age 13)

I am a special education teacher at my daughter Elizabeth's school. Our school has a team approach to transitioning students with special needs. During the first day of school, the teacher assistant meets with the students and assists them in getting their lockers open, getting to class on time, organizing schoolwork, and helping with assignments. In the afternoon the autism teacher conducts a social skills study class. It gives the students a break in their day where they can relax and be themselves. The teacher assistant also works on organization of notebooks, homework, decision-making skills, social interactions, as well as hall issues, lunch issues, and other daily problems. With the support of our team, all eight of our ASD students have had a successful start of the school year. My daughter, Elizabeth, benefits greatly from this approach and is enjoying middle school life.

Elizabeth's school team has done a wonderful job in preparing her for the transition to middle school. All school teams can follow these simple steps to creating a successful transition plan. Some of the steps may take some time, but a proactive approach will prevent problem behaviors and will benefit the young woman with ASD.

Conclusion

The elementary and middle school years are a time of acquiring new knowledge, learning new skills, overcoming obstacles, and preparing for high school and beyond. Parents and professionals should seek training and ongoing support to fully understand the many complexities of ASD. The multidisciplinary team, which includes general education teachers, special education teachers, speech-language pathologists, occupational therapists, school psychologists, administrators, and the parents, must collaborate and share their expertise in order to create a positive learning environment for girls with ASD. The team should plan ongoing proactive meetings to reduce problems and communicate proactive strategies for planning for the future.

CHAPTER 4

Adolescence and Early Adulthood

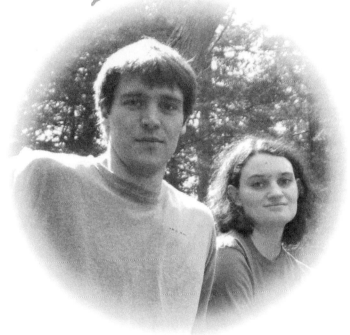

"What's a French kiss?"
Mattie, age 11

"You don't have to worry about that right now.
Wait until you are 16 to ask me."
Danielle, Mattie's mom

*T*his is a typical question from a young adolescent girl with ASD. All young women experience myriad questions and challenges during adolescence, including appearance, personal hygiene, dating, and puberty. Thus, although a young adolescent like Mattie may have a developmental delay, her physical development continues to progress similarly to that of typically developing girls. Her social maturity may be limited, but her physical changes and growth will continue throughout adolescence, which can pose challenges and insecurity for any young woman and her family.

In this chapter, we will discuss puberty, personal hygiene, dating, self-determination, and gender identity. Adolescent girls with ASD will provide insight into their world as teenagers. Building independent skills such as self-determination and self-advocacy will be discussed. The chapter will also review current trends in transitioning from high school, employment challenges, and post-secondary training. Finally, we offer advice and input from other parents and adult women with ASD with regard to the future.

Adolescence is a period when school yard discussions turn to boys, clothing styles, and sexuality. TV, music, and the media send powerful images that push young women to adulthood and to question their appearance, their bodies, and their relationships. These images can ultimately affect a young women's self-esteem (Fine & Asch, 1988).

Parents, like Danielle, are not always prepared to handle new questions about oncoming puberty and the opposite sex. The topic of adolescence and puberty is vast. This chapter will focus on the most salient issues regarding young women with ASD.

Beauty Is Only Skin Deep

By Karen (Mother of Rosemarie, age 17)

I worried about Rosemarie going through puberty and tried to plan ahead for some of the issues she would face. At the bookstore, I happened upon the American Girl Library of books dealing with girls' issues. We started with The Care and Keeping of You – The Body Book for Girls. *I can't praise this book enough for the wonderful guide that it is and how it helped explain a whole range of body and health basics. We then added* The Care and Keeping of Me – The Body Book Journal, Oops! The Manners Guide for Girls, The Feelings Book – The Care and Keeping of Your Emotions, The Care and Keeping of Friends, Help! An Indispensable Guide to Life For Girls! *and* Yikes! A Smart Girls Guide to Surviving Tricky, Sticky, Icky Situations. *The titles alone attracted me to these books, which are written in a simple style, with humor and sensitivity. Rosemarie is a very visual thinker, and the illustrations are great for the visual learner. Since we first started using these books, when Rosemarie was around age 10, she has read them over and over and still uses them as references.*

Rosemarie is like any other young woman, interested in learning about her body and puberty. Our society places an enormous amount of focus on appearance. According to Rousso and Wehmeyer (2002), an attractive appearance for a young woman in our society is linked to intelligence, kindness, and overall influence. Yet, young women with ASD may be ambivalent about appearance and personal hygiene. "Girls with ASD may not see the value in their appearance. They may decide to wear comfortable clothing and not like to care for their personal hygiene" (Attwood, 1999). Their decisions on what clothing to wear may be influenced by their sensory needs or by their need for repetition and consistency rather than the latest fashion fad.

By Kimberly Tucker

From *Women from Another Planet* (2003)

It was fifth grade. I loved my white sweater; so very soft to the touch, like a rabbit. I needed comforting things. The other kids would mention "you wear that sweater every day. Don't you have any other clothes?" Of course I had other clothes – probably wore that sweater all year, every day. (p. 131)

Kimberly is typical of young women with ASD, unaware of some of the societal rules about appearance and clothing. She represents many young women with ASD who struggle to "fit in." Temple Grandin has reported on her experiences with wearing certain clothing, "During the highly social years of middle and high school, dressing outside the norm will make you the subject of teasing and bullying, absolutely and always ... Trouble arises because Aspies themselves do not place much importance on what they wear and how they look and consequently they don't pay attention to hygiene, they dress like a slob or wear mismatched clothes or clothes that don't fit. Whenever I see an Aspie peer who is doing that I get right on them" (Grandin, 2005, p. 314).

Dr. Grandin makes an important point about how we can support young women during this period. We must point out these hidden rules and provide young women with the tools to make good decisions about their appearance. Zosia Zaks (2006) explains:

> Men and women are judged differently when it comes to personal appearance. While the world often tolerates a little sloppiness from men, women are under pressure to look attractive. Hundreds of magazines and tons of media bandwidth are devoted to hair, make-up, color, style, and fashion for women. Men who appear grungy, archaic in their fashion sense, or just eccentric are usually excused for this shortcoming. It is assumed that such a guy works in a messy occupation, doesn't have a girlfriend to fix him up, or is just – simply put – being a guy. But a grungy, unkempt, or strange-looking woman is a spectacle. Even in casual circles women feel pressured to look a certain way. Women on the spectrum who cannot or choose not to put themselves together in a way society expects are often viewed as childish, disorderly, or rebellious and not accorded respect or taken seriously. (p. 301)

Clothing is only one part of a person's appearance. Adequate personal hygiene is another important aspect. Parents may struggle with their daughter to maintain appropriate personal hygiene during adolescence. Daily tasks of washing, brushing, and grooming are critical for peer acceptance, yet may not be a priority for young women with ASD (Bashe & Kirby, 2001). As with appearance, your daughter may not understand the nuances of personal hygiene and how they impact social relationships and future outcomes.

Body changes, growth, and menstruation are just a few of the developmental milestones that will occur for all young women beginning around age 10 (Shaw, 1999). Certain hormones increase during adolescence, causing both physical and emotional changes. As mentioned, hormones can cause moodiness, anxiety, weight gain or loss, angry outbursts, and drops in self-esteem (Gurian, 2002). These are no less evident in young women with ASD.

By April Masilamani

From *Women from Another Planet* (2003)

My physical development was also a shock. Although I had been given a talk by my mother, it was an explanation from a medical textbook and I could talk knowledgeably about progesterone and such, but had made no connection between the information and what was happening to my body. (p. 145)

April provides us with an important message for all parents and professionals working with young women with ASD: We must provide information that is visual, practical, and readily applicable to a given situation. There are several strategies to follow in supporting young women with ASD during this challenging period.

1. **Start early.** Begin communicating about puberty at an early age. Books from the library can be great resources, but in addition to presenting the facts, parents and professionals must provide practical application to the girl's current situation. Start slowly and provide practical information in small amounts.

2. **Practice.** Some young women with ASD experience sensory problems and may have difficulty with such items as a new bra or sanitary napkins. Try several types for a short while, even before it is necessary.

By Karen (Mother of Rosemarie, age 17)

Just before Rosemarie started her period, I read a magazine article about making a girl's first period fun. This was certainly a new concept to me! Send her flowers, prepare a special dinner, or buy her something pretty. So this is what we did. Also, every so often, I would have Rosemarie wear a pad for a little while to get her used to the feel of it before the actual event occurred.

3. **Select teachable moments.** It is not enough to just have "the talk." Teaching about body changes, menstruation, and sexuality must occur on a regular basis and in teachable moments. For example, if you notice your daughter sprouting underarm hair, it is time to talk about shaving and using deodorant.

4. **Create a daily personal hygiene checklist.** Using visuals, develop a checklist, either handwritten or on the computer, that includes the tasks required each day to maintain appropriate personal hygiene. This would include: brush teeth for 2 minutes, wash hair with shampoo, select clean clothes, apply deodorant, and comb hair. The daily checklist allows the young woman to be more independent but still gives her direction.

5. **Review public vs. private.** As discussed in the section on social skills objectives, specific rules dictate public vs. private

information. We must let our young women know who they can turn to for honest answers about their development and when it is appropriate to ask questions. For example, Mattie needs to know that it is O.K. to ask Mom about French kissing but not the custodian at school.

6. **Build self-advocacy skills.** Self-awareness and advocacy will be further discussed later in this chapter. It is important to know that a young woman with a positive self-image and strong advocacy skills will develop into a more independent adult woman (Rousso & Wehmeyer, 2002).

Beauty may be only skin deep, but our culture will judge young women based on their personal hygiene and appearance. Parents and professionals should explicitly teach the required skills for acceptable personal hygiene and appearance but also support their independence and uniqueness. Young women with ASD need a loving support system when tiptoeing through the mine field of adolescence and puberty.

Gender Issues: Boys vs. Girls

Puberty, appearance, and personal hygiene are just a few of the ongoing challenges for young women with ASD. Many women with ASD report experiencing issues regarding gender identity. Most girls, by age 11, have developed gender identity. That is, a girl knows she's a girl and begins to relate to other girls differently than to boys (Gurian, 2002). But this type of relating to other females may be delayed or non-existent for some type of young women with ASD.

By Jane Meyerding

From *Women from Another Planet* (2003)

When I say I don't feel like a woman, people are likely to assume that I mean I feel like a man. I don't. Never have — never learned to see my body as a woman's body in the sense that a woman's body is an actor in socio-sexual relations. My body is the support structure for me, my intellect, my memories, my sensory experiences. If it has a gender, that gender lives on the outside, not in here where it would make a difference to how I feel or see the world (except that in so far as I am shaped by how my gender causes the world to see and feel about me). (p. 157)

Jane helps us to understand that stereotyping by gender can be very limiting. Here again, our society and the media force images upon us based on how women are supposed to look and behave. For example, all women are to be nurturing and empathetic. As a gender, women are supposed to be motherly, docile, and passive. Men are allowed much more latitude for being self-centered and aloof. Many young women with ASD may appear to have more male-like characteristics, which consequently can separate them from bonding with other females (Zaks, 2006).

This conflict with gender identity can have a negative impact on the developing self-esteem (Lonsdale, 1997). If young women with ASD do not feel they are fulfilling their female role, this can result in "high rates of low self-esteem, depression, and anxiety" (Zaks, 2006, p. 298). Self-image and identity are intrinsically linked. Young women with ASD may not conform to the unspoken social rules and hidden expectations that often appear illogical to them.

By Jane Meyerding

From *Women from Another Planet* (2003)

When people perceive me as aloof, they are sensing an absence of emotional availability. It is unwomanly of me, in traditional terms, to be the way I am. In feminist terms, it is unsisterly. I just have to accept that. For this autistic, it's normal. (p. 169)

With the combination of limiting gender identity and its impact on self-esteem, parents and professionals must focus on the strengths of young women with ASD. At no time is this more important than during adolescence.

According to Rousso and Wehmeyer (2002), we must:

- Challenge our thoughts on gender and stereotypes
- Provide opportunities to build on existing skills
- Educate and advocate; knowledge is power
- Encourage problem-solving skills
- Open ourselves up to a different way of thinking

Young women with ASD can build lives that are not subjected to narrow-minded stereotypes with an appropriate amount of support, understanding, and education. We must have high expectations that they will develop personal relationships that might not reflect traditional roles. Through self-determination, advocacy, and networking with the community, young women with ASD can have highly successful lives that will allow them to live independently, create close personal relationships, and maintain fulfilling employment.

Who Am I?
Self-Determination

By Karen (Mother of Rosemarie, age 17)

Rosemarie is in her last year of high school. She has faithfully kept up with all the required subjects; she reads and writes well and is a talented artist, which I am extremely proud of. Is she now ready to go on? Physically and intellectually, Rosemarie is a "normal" 17-year-old. Most of the time she acts and reacts much younger, socially and emotionally, however. How does a parent handle a teen given such circumstances? How do I prepare her for a life of independence? Here I am, in one moment answering questions about sex and world events and a moment later trying to divert a temper tantrum that rivals that of a toddler, over an issue that would concern only a toddler.

It seems that most areas of Rosemarie's life present such challenges. Her artwork is wonderful and she draws all the time, effortlessly. But, ask her to draw something for you, and suddenly the pressure is too much for her to handle. The same applies to her writing. Rosemarie expresses herself very well in writing, and has deep insight into herself and her autism. The same is true for cooking, exercising, going places, you name it. She enjoys much in life, and she has much to share with the world, but only on her terms. I have learned that if you push her, just even a little, she shuts down. As a proud parent with high aspirations for both my sons and Rosemarie, it has been painful over the years for me to try to resist my passionate urges to motivate, guide, persuade, beg – whatever I felt necessary – to move her toward what I perceived (or what others suggested) as an important goal. But have I been nearsighted in my efforts to help her be "all that she can be"? "Now what?" I ask myself.

As a parent, Karen is torn between guiding her daughter through adolescence and allowing her the independence to find her own path. With the onset of puberty and the changes in physical appearance and questions about gender identity that go with it, we are often caught in a quagmire between too much and too little support. This is true for all young people, but especially so for girls on the autism spectrum. The future for young women with ASD is compromised by bias and stereotyping, which we must counteract by fostering and supporting self-determination and independence and allowing them to be "all that they can be." There are several steps that Karen and other families can take to increase independence and self-advocacy.

Self-Advocacy

Self-advocacy is part of the process towards self-determination. It involves educating and empowering individuals with disabilities to advocate for their own needs and determine their own destiny. Appropriate advocacy skills allow young women with ASD to understand their value as persons and future opportunities. Self-determination is not limited by societal standards and traditional roles. According to Hall, Kleinert, and Kearns (2000), students who have become empowered with self-determination skills have more successful post-school outcomes. Further research suggests that students who are empowered with self-determination skills have higher rates of employment and earn a higher wage one year after graduation than students who do not (Test, Karvonen, Wood, Browder, & Algozzine, 2000; Wehmeyer & Schwartz, 1997).

By Lynley (Mother of Jazz, age 16)

From *Autism Is Not a Life Sentence* (2005)

Jessica [Jazz] knew from about age 6 that she had autism, and she understood to the extent a 6-year-old can what it meant to be autistic. I had to educate myself about all the ways Autism affects the brain and how it affects the processing of information. Then it was my job to pass my learning onto Jessica in a positive and constructive way. I knew that attitude would be the key to unleashing and nurturing Jessica's full potential. Perception is the key. I told her that it was important that she understand that some kids have freckles because they have sensitive skin. Some kids wear eyeglasses because their eyes don't work like yours and mine do. Some kids have blonde hair and some have black hair. Some have autism, and some kids are afraid of the dark; some are in wheelchairs, some have legs that work just fine, some kids like grape jelly and some others don't like jelly at all with their peanut butter — that's just the way it is. It's neither good nor bad.

She listened and took all this in, and then nodded. It made sense to us both. As long as we didn't make a big deal out of it, then it shouldn't BE a big deal. The main point that I

*made to Jessica was that having autism was an explanation
for why things seemed out of place to her sometimes or why
she might feel out of control at times, but never, ever, was it
to be used as an excuse for why she couldn't do something. If
anything, it should be the opposite. We used autism to motivate her. She and I agreed that autism or not, she wouldn't
limit herself. (p. 7)*

To begin the journey of self-determination, young women must
acquire accurate knowledge about their disability. Jessica's mother
decided when Jessica was still at an early age to be open and positive about her disability. This is the first step in self-determination. Young women with ASD experience an invisible disability.
That is, they may appear to be fully functioning and typically
developing in certain environments and under certain circumstances, but a change in the schedule or a challenge to their sensory system can cause increased symptoms and atypical behaviors
to appear. It is difficult for society to accept a disability that they
cannot visually observe (Hoffschmidt & Weinstein, 2003). Thus,
they can easily misinterpret behaviors and assume the individual
with ASD is being lazy, unorganized, or rude, for example.

In addition, according to Zosia Zaks (2006), "in general, girls and
women have a much greater tendency to become depressed or withdrawn when upset. For this reason, the extent of a woman's frustra-
tions and limitations may not be readily apparent" (p. 293).

The challenge for young women with ASD is to first understand themselves and then to be able to adequately explain their
strengths and limitations to future employers, friends, and college
professors. Parents and professionals can assist young women in
the process by:

- Providing them with facts and resources about autism and Asperger Syndrome
- Defining terms and behavioral symptoms associated with ASD
- Identifying appropriate special education programs
- Focusing on their strengths
- Developing specific techniques for dealing with behavioral limitations
- Discussing the disability openly and frequently as they develop through adolescence
- Role-playing new-found advocacy skills

We must continue to communicate the positive aspects of the disability and can learn from Jessica and her mother. Not only must we provide the facts and resources about ASD, we must also discuss the limitations associated with the disability. It is only through this realization that our young women can truly self-advocate for their needs and future goals. In the next story, Jazz shares how she is setting her own goals and taking pride in her accomplishments.

By Jazz (age 16 with ASD)

The goals that my mom set for me are attainable, and lots of them I've hurdled already. I set even more goals for myself. At the end of my sophomore year, I was inducted into the National Honor Society. On the day of the induction at Mills, my mom, "the rooster mother," was so proud. My family was there for the ceremony, and we took a picture which actually made it into the Arkansas Times *magazine, because it was of four generations of women in our family to be in National Honor Soci-*

ety. Nobody ever dreamed when I started school, in a preschool handicap program in North Carolina where they suggested that I wear a helmet, that this day would be possible.

Self-Determination and the IEP

Although the importance of self-determination for young women with ASD is widely recognized, the IEP does not always reflect long-term goals in this area. Therefore, it is important that the IEP team, including the young woman with ASD, address the goals and objectives for self-determination, which include knowledge about the disability, self-awareness, goal setting, and self-advocacy.

Educating young women with ASD about their disability must include a discussion about disclosure of the disability. Should she tell her peers? What about employers? Who can she tell and how?

Disclosure is a very personal decision between the young woman and her parents. Disclosure means more than just telling someone "I have ASD." It can result in negative outcomes. Discrimination against people with disabilities still exists, and young women with ASD should prepare themselves for a variety of reactions to disclosure of their disability. Negative responses from peers or teachers may discourage them from sharing in the future and should be addressed by the team.

By Liane Holliday Willey

From *Pretending to Be Normal* (1999)

Despite my belief in full disclosure, I will admit there are many times I wish I had never mentioned the words "Asperger's Syndrome." I have met with some very real prejudices and some very painful misunderstandings on several occasions when I have tried to explain to strangers, friends, and even family members what life with AS is like. I wish I could say I understood their reluctance to be open, empathetic and caring, for if I did, I would find peace. But, I cannot. I fill with anger each time I recall the reactions that have left me cold, frustrated, furious, embarrassed or worse, ashamed of who I am. (p. 125)

Several strategies may be implemented to help minimize the experiences and frustration shared by Liane Holliday Willey. Detailed preparation must be part of the training for a young woman with ASD about who, when, and how to disclose her disability.

- Create a list of people who should be informed about her disability, including teachers and employers.
- Develop another list of people who may not need to know; friends at school or church group members, for example.
- Role-play how and when to disclose information about ASD.
- Part of the role-play should include using "I" statements, appropriate nonverbal gestures, and assertive speech patterns (Lynch & Gussel, 1996).

- Prepare and role-play specific responses to potential negative remarks.
- Create and write out a short description of the disability with strengths and needs.
- Develop a short list of references and resources to accompany the disclosure.

Even though disclosure may lead to some negative outcomes, it can provide benefits to young women with ASD. Allowing them to advocate for their own needs empowers them to accept their strengths and needs and to plan for the future accordingly.

Some adolescents have difficulty accepting their limitations. There may be periods when they are in denial of the limitations associated with their disability while developing skills for self-advocacy and disclosure. Self-determination must include making honest self-appraisals, which may include identifying weaknesses.

By Stephanie (Mother of Gianna, age 15)

Gianna is 15 and was diagnosed with Asperger Syndrome five years ago. As any typical adolescent, she does not want to be singled out among her peers. She is quite conscientious about "fitting in." During her last IEP meeting, Gianna refused to accept speech services. She did not want to be pulled out of class to receive speech therapy. The rest of the team went along with her decision, and the speech therapist remains on a consultation basis one time per month for the general education teachers.

Gianna's decision to stop speech therapy was part of a typical teenager's unwillingness to stand out from the crowd and acknowledge that she needs help. This can be frustrating for both parents and professionals, but the IEP team must acknowledge the student's rights to make decisions about her needs. As part of the self-determination process, we must provide opportunities for developing decision-making skills. In this case, the team must review the goals of speech therapy and balance them against Gianna's wishes.

Self-determination places the decision making and control in the hands of the young women with a disability. This encourages creative problem solving and ways to examine options. Can Gianna receive speech therapy after school? Or can the speech therapist consult with her general education teachers to develop strategies to be included in the classroom? While self-determination will ultimately give the young woman control over her own destiny, especially early on, it can be frightening to parents and professionals.

Networking and Community Outreach

Young women with ASD need opportunities to successfully interact with the world. Sometimes this is difficult in typical social situations due to their challenges in the area of social skills. Networking with others with disabilities can be very beneficial in building self-determination as well as self-confidence. As discussed under social skills development, the need for planned opportunities as steps towards independence and friendship making continues throughout adulthood.

Parents and professionals must play an active role in creating these opportunities. Review websites and community support groups to find an appropriate match. Model this behavior yourself by joining a support group and talking to others who have children with disabilities. Also, look for opportunities to attend autism or Asperger Syndrome workshops or conferences in your area. Finding out that there are other young women like herself, with similar feelings, concerns, and experiences, can help decrease your daughter's sense of isolation and support her future endeavors. If such opportunities are not available locally, explore chat and on-line discussion groups run for and by individuals with ASD.

Young women with ASD need opportunities to experience membership in community organizations or school groups. Encourage participation in and help to identify extracurricular groups, such as small social clubs, recreation groups, or church activities, that might have similar interests and talents.

Select groups that are highly supervised and structured. Be sure to visit the group first to be sure your daughter has the skills to be successful and that members share her interests and talents. Identify what social skills may be necessary and address them at home. Joining a carefully chosen (based on interests and ability level) community group will help to increase the young woman's feelings of self-worth by focusing on her talents and strengths.

Part of networking should also include identifying positive role models within the disability community. Luckily, due to the pioneering efforts of many talented women with ASD who have come forward to share their stories, many resources are available for young women with ASD to learn what others like themselves have experienced and achieved.

According to NICHCY (www.nichcy.org), there are several ways to expose young women with disabilities to positive role models.

- From early childhood onward, seek out women with similar disabilities in your community who are working, raising families, and doing the things that most women do. Invite them to your daughter's school or arrange for your daughter to meet with these women and hear them share their experiences.

- Acquaint your daughter with the world of work from an early age. Talk to her about a variety of jobs and have high expectations. Do this in a way that conveys that many career paths are open to her. ASD girls can be successful in caring for animals (veterinary clinics, animal shelters), volunteering at senior citizen organizations and hospitals, and tutoring younger children. Many are budding artists and may be able to put their talents to use in related areas.

- Be sure the school has a good selection of learning materials about people with disabilities. Check to make sure they are not presented in stereotypical female and male roles. Become active in helping your child's teacher locate resources.

Exposing young women with ASD to positive role models can help them see the possibilities for a bright future. Self-determination should begin early in the child's development. Focusing on strengths, encouraging problem-solving skills, and disability awareness can begin in elementary school. As the young woman matures, her level of self-determination will change and increase. Being active in extracurricular activities, meeting role models, and networking with other women will provide positive outcomes, including higher rates of long-term employment.

Transition Planning

A large part of planning for future independence will take place during transition meetings with the school. Three significant laws help to govern transition planning for students with ASD. According to the IDEA, if a young woman with ASD has an IEP and receives special education services through the school district, the school team must create a transition plan by the time she is 16. Further, beyond school age, the Americans with Disabilities Act (ADA) and Section 504 of the Vocational Rehabilitation Act provide protections for employment and educational programs into adulthood.

Information on IDEA, Section 504, or ADA

www.wrightslaw.com/info/sec504.summ.rights.htm

www.ed.gov/about/offices/list/ocr/qa-disability..html

www.ed.gov/about/offices/list/ocr/504faq.html

www.ed.gov/about/offices/list/ocr/docs/edlite-FAPE504.html

Individual Transition Plan (ITP)

Most school teams begin the transition planning process when students are 14 years of age. The ITP is designed to map out the future for students with disabilities. According to Reed Martin (2003), a special education attorney, the transition planning process is a time to evaluate existing programs and services to determine how they are preparing a student for life after school.

As stipulated by the IDEA, the ITP must address the following:

- Postsecondary education
- Vocational training
- Integrated or supportive employment
- Continuing and adult education
- Adult services
- Independent living
- Community participation

There is a great need for intensive transition planning for young women with disabilities. Rousso and Wehmeyer (2002) found a gender gap between males and females with disabilities. Males with disabilities are more likely to have employment post-high school than females with disabilities, and women with disabilities who were employed were working in unskilled jobs. In addition, being a white, older male with a disability was linked to a higher probability of competitive employment. This research supports the need for parents, professionals, and young women with ASD themselves to work together to create a transition plan that will assist in developing independence and preparedness for successful adult outcomes.

IEP Meeting

Attending an IEP meeting can be an overwhelming experience for the adolescent. Parents and professionals should prepare the student for attending a transition meeting. Both teachers and parents can implement the following strategies for creating a positive IEP meeting.

- Review the transition document before the meeting

- Assess the young woman's specific strengths and interests
- Create a draft copy of the transition plan
- Identify who will be attending the meeting
- Role-play attending the meeting and review what will be discussed
- Develop a list of questions she may want to ask of the team
- Prepare any materials she may want to bring to the meeting
- Review problem-solving skills that may be necessary during the meeting

Attending the transition meeting will empower the student with the knowledge and decision-making skills that she will need for the future. This will allow her to advocate for herself and to effectively communicate her goals.

By Temple Grandin

From *Unwritten Rules of Social Relationships* (2005)

Kids with ASD need a lot of preparation and training, training that needs to be part of elementary, middle, and high school education if they're going to have any kind of life after they get out of school. (p. 46)

Dr. Grandin's assertions are correct. With proper planning and supports, adults with ASD are capable of supporting themselves and living independent, enriching lives. Developing a successful transition plan will help ensure this goal. Successful transition planning must be student-centered, goal-oriented, and present a comprehensive vision for the future.

Student-Centered

It is imperative that young women with ASD be included in the IEP process when developing the transition plan. This principle follows the guidelines discussed for self-determination and self-advocacy. It is based on the student's strengths, preferences, and interests.

The school team, parents, and the young woman with ASD can begin by asking questions about what she likes to do and what her of areas interest are. Review any extracurricular activities and hobbies as possible future employment opportunities (Grandin & Duffy, 2004). Assess for weaknesses as well as strengths and plan for obstacles. For example, she may have volunteered at the veterinary hospital. Her areas of weakness were cleaning the cages and answering the phone, but she excelled at walking and grooming the animals. In this case, the team needs to continue training on phone and cleaning skills.

Work with the school team to identify employment opportunities that will target the young woman's areas of interests and validate her strengths. On the following page, Ashley explains some of her strengths and weaknesses that should be discussed during transition planning.

By Ashley (age 20 with ASD)

Another Asperger tendency that I noticed during these years was my inability to play sports. I attempted tennis, softball, and basketball, but my motor skills seemed to be lacking. I had hand-eye coordination issues with the ball, and I discovered in my first season of basketball that I could not jump and catch the ball at the same time. It was either one or the other.

Soon after this, I started playing the flute in a marching band, and became quite good at memorizing my music and places on the field. I played and marched at the same time without any difficulties, and I soon became one of the best marchers in band. This is probably because marching band is all about repetition; we continually practiced the same music and the same movements, so there were few surprises. On the other hand, in basketball, you can try to plan certain plays, but if the other team doesn't comply, you have to come up with a new strategy on the spot. I seemed to have quite a bit of trouble in that area. I have never been quick on my feet.

Goal-Oriented

The transition plan must outline specific goals to be addressed during high school and into adulthood. The team, including the student with disabilities, should identify long-range goals with a coordinated set of activities that are assigned to team members and include a timeline. These activities might include further vocational training, structured community experiences, and instruction in daily living skills. Interagency collaboration with the Department of Vocational Rehabilitation will also be part of the transition plan. Representatives from Voc Rehab may attend the meetings and assist the team in identifying community supports.

Comprehensive Vision for the Future

The heart of the ITP is a vision for the future. Young women with ASD need a transition plan that will allow them to attain the highest possible level of achievement and success. Parents and professionals should have high expectations and not be limited by stereotypes and skepticism. The transition plan will evolve over time and take new directions as the young woman moves through high school and learns new skills. At its core, the ITP should be a working document that assists young women with ASD in achieving their goals and living and working independently.

Young women with ASD face a myriad roadblocks when planning for the future and living independently. For example, an employer may have a false belief that a woman with a disability cannot work a full-time job or that she should not be paid the same as a nondisabled individual. Sadly, certain stereotypes, employment gaps, and gender bias can greatly impact future opportunities (Rousso & Wehmeyer, 2001).

As parents and professionals we can teach our young women with ASD to achieve to the greatest extent of their capability. We must allow them to succeed in living independently, if appropriate, through self-determination and proper transition planning. According to Zosia Zaks (2006), "When you live by yourself, the obvious advantage is that you do not have to deal with anybody else. ... Having total control over your environment can provide relief" (p. 61).

Positive future outcomes require planning, preparation, and a collaborative effort among school, home, and community agencies. In order to live independently, a young woman needs to be able to handle financial responsibilities, utilize transportation, shop for basic necessities, and respond to emergency situations, among other things. Because women with disabilities often face two powerful stereotypes – helplessness and dependency – parents and professionals must believe that young women with ASD can achieve, work, and live independently (Resources for Rehabilitation, 1994).

The Dating Game

By Liane Holliday Willey

From *Pretending to Be Normal* (1999)

The men I had been dating were nice men who shared some of my interests and hobbies, but with each of them there was always an unspoken and unseen something that stood between us – like that curtain that kept the truth of the Wizard from the people of OZ. I never gave much thought to what the curtain was hiding because when I did, it led me to distraction. (p. 78)

Dating is a difficult developmental stage for any young woman. Young women with ASD have an even more difficult time understanding the complexities of the opposite sex and how to maneuver the dating world (Zaks, 2006). Learning the idiosyncrasies of males and how to read their body language and thoughts is a struggle shared by many girls in their teenage years. Dating may be delayed based on the young woman's level of maturity. Families may have certain rules and expectations for dating. Some parents may feel pressure to have their daughter start dating, whereas others may want to protect and shelter her. Families should wait until their daughter feels confident in her skills before embarking on the dating scene.

Although dating may not be directly a school issue, it is discussed by teachers and counselors, and school personnel should be involved with teaching appropriate social skills for adolescents, including peer tutors. Therefore, it is important that both family members and school staff have a clear understanding of how to support the adolescent girl with ASD during this challenging time. Remember that all individuals seek loving relationships and will benefit from our guidance, as Jana explains in her story.

By Jana (age 27 with ASD)

After my last relationship ended, I took an extended leave of absence from the dating game. I spent almost two years by myself, strengthening my character by developing the communication skills and patience I needed to succeed. The emotional maturity I gained through this experience allowed me to recognize exactly what I wanted and needed in a partner. I met my husband-to-be at a bookstore in the math section, which is not at all shocking. We hit it off immediately. It was then I decided that happiness meant more to me than knowing a million factoids. Because I made a decision to grow emotionally, my ability to memorize large quantities of information, among other things, became affected. I struggled with feelings of intellectual inadequacy because I could no longer remember things I'd previously learned. Although this created a gap between my former "logical" self and the newly minted "girlie" persona, my learning experience has been deeply enriched by my newfound ability to associate emotions with information. Best of all, my husband appreciates the sacrifices I've made to improve myself, and I finally know how it feels to be in a real loving relationship.

The first challenge a young woman with ASD may encounter is understanding the difference between friends who are boys and boyfriends. Adults should concretely explain that boys may just want to be friends without dating. A boyfriend spends more time with you alone, share hobbies or other interests, calls you at home, or compliments you repeatedly. Discuss these specific behaviors beginning in elementary school and more often in adolescence. This is another example of the importance of knowing the "hidden curriculum" for behavior. As mentioned earlier, *The Hidden Curriculum* (2004) by Myles, Trautman, and Schelvan is a great resource for teaching these skills.

Second, parents and other concerned adults should begin to teach specific dating behaviors. It is important to not assume that your daughter has the skills to interact appropriately with boys. Talk openly and provide specific strategies for dealing with such issues.

For example,

- Suggest topics to discuss: movies, TV, pets, school, and family.
- Practice and role-play at home. Have your daughter pretend she is talking to a boy and give her feedback on voice tone, nonverbal skills, physical proximity, and eye contact. Create short scenarios that may occur on a date and rehearse what to say in difficult moments.
- Have your daughter work on giving specific age-appropriate compliments.
- Make a list with your daughter of appropriate things to do and where to go. Brainstorm together and write them down: bowling, eating out, movies, going to the mall, athletic activities.
- Make a list of activities not to engage in:
  - Being alone in the park
  - Walking in new places
  - Driving too far from home
  - Going some place you have never been before
  - Going to a place that was not on the schedule

All adolescent girls experience some level of anxiety and nervousness when dating. Zosia Zaks (2006) shares her insights on dating, "When it comes to dating and romance, one problem for autistic adults can be society's expectations. It seems like everybody knows how to follow some secret "script" – except those of us on the spectrum. Yet, while it may appear as if other people know exactly what to do when it comes to dating, everyone is just as confused, scared, and excited as you are" (p. 183).

For young women with ASD, the anxiety levels may increase due to the novelty of the experience, change in routines, and some of the sensory challenges involved in meeting a new person. A simple date of dinner and a movie can create challenges with eating some place new, traveling to new places, and being in large crowds.

Adults can help minimize anxiety by setting limits or rules for dating. Create family rules for dating that address acceptable age for dating, meeting the boy prior to dating, how long a date should last, and similar guidelines that are compatible with your family's values and your daughter's needs. These boundaries will assist your daughter in feeling safe and less anxious.

Another tool for easing anxiety is developing a checklist for dates:

- Check your clothes and hygiene.
- Review topics of interests for discussion and conversation starters.
- Stay on the designated schedule for departure and arriving home.
- Review levels of appropriate touching.
- Review the safety plan (see p. 190).
- Have fun.

Young women with ASD experience delays in many areas of their social development, including dating. This type of checklist will help guide them through the dating process.

Safety Concerns

According to Dennis Debbault (2003), girls with ASD are at heightened risk for sexual assault and date rape. Similarly, the

National Center for Injury Prevention and Control (1998) reported that students with disabilities are at a greater risk for sexual harassment than nondisabled peers because they are often seen as targets who will not be believed if they report the harassment (Rousso & Wehmeyer, 2001).

This pattern of harassment is similar to the characteristics of bullying discussed earlier. Girls with ASD may miss the signs of aggression or misunderstand a boy's affection. Therefore, adults should concretely explain the signs of harassment and assault.

By Jana (age 27 with ASD)

Maneuvering through the mine field of everyday existence was a piece of cake compared to grasping the concept of love. Finding sexual partners did not pose a challenge to me; however, creating mutually gratifying relationships proved to be nearly impossible. Unfortunately, most of my knowledge of how to act in a relationship came from my exposure to Hollywood's nonstop parade of sexual affairs through watching movies and reading gossip publications. This distorted perspective deprived me of a healthy sexual connection until my mid 20s. Although I desperately wanted to be in a loving relationship, I had an extremely difficult time understanding the concept of intimacy. Sex was always mechanical, and an orgasm seemed entirely out of reach because I had no idea of how to attain an orgasm.

Jana had opportunities to find sexual partners, and this included some difficult experiences. Parents and professionals working with young women with ASD must assist them in developing a safe dating environment. In this connection, it is important to create a safety plan, which would include the following:

- Identify appropriate levels of affection: hand holding or short periods of hugging.
- Role-play nonverbal communication skills that are age-appropriate: physical proximity, where to touch, ways to flirt appropriately, and so on.
- Create a safety word for her to use to discreetly end the date. For example, she can call home and say "Puppy," which is the key word for ending the date. This will alert her parents that she is having a problem on the date, and they can make immediate arrangement to pick her up.
- Role-play how to deal with a young man's anger. For example, if a young man seems angry, diffuse the situation by saying you are not feeling well and need to go home.
- Write out a list of cell phone numbers to call in an emergency.
- Review the steps for preventing bullying by remaining in public places, verbalizing a strong response to a harassment attempt, and having an escape plan.

These simple steps can support the young woman during the date and help prevent an escalation of harassment. Many teenage girls do not recognize the early signs and may not fully understand the rules for safe dating. Adults should also be familiar with the signs of an abusive relationship and be prepared to discuss this topic with young woman (Rousso & Wehmeyer, 2001).

Signs can include the following:

- He checks on her too much.
- He is obsessed with her whereabouts.
- He shows up unannounced to spot check.

- She seems afraid of him.
- You overhear him call her names.
- He is overly moody.
- He does not want to spend time with your family.

Just a Reminder

Harassment can occur over the computer, too. Parents should be sure to follow these rules for Internet access:

1. Tell their daughter not to spend too much time online.

2. Monitor chat rooms and Internet history.

3. Teach their daughter to keep certain information private.

4. Review e-mail conversations.

Dating can be a challenging period for your daughter and the family, but with the right supports and boundaries, it can be a time for growth and independence. Although there are safety concerns when a young woman starts dating, parents must resist the temptation to restrict her independence and keep her at home. Restricting access to social situations and experiences will have negative consequences and limit her ability to distinguish different types of relationships and ultimately create a sense of social isolation. With the appropriate supports and teaching opportunities, most young women with ASD can experience a wide range of social relationships and enjoy the dating process. Encourage positive interactions with structure and boundaries.

College

By Charlotte (age 32 with ASD)

I received my bachelor's degree from a prestigious university in suburban Boston. It was a purely academic college, which was perfect for me. I could lose myself in my studies. Once I got involved in student clubs where I had to work in team-like situations, my Asperger's came out. For example, when I became secretary of the Student Senate, I was expected to transcribe the minutes of the weekly meetings. Once I printed them out, they were to be approved at the next meeting. When the minutes were criticized by the other Senate members at the next meeting, I didn't see why I had to make the approved changes. The other students on the Senate weren't very nice to me once this happened, and I couldn't understand why. Somebody would have had to show me the appropriate way to conduct myself.

Charlotte has highlighted both the positive and the negative experiences that many young women with ASD encounter in college. Although she enjoyed the academic studies, she was not prepared for the social demands. While all young women with ASD will not go to college like Charlotte, it is within the reach of many. If a young woman with ASD has the basic academic competence, she can successfully attend postsecondary education with reasonable accommodations (Lynch & Gussel, 1996).

Parents and professionals can prepare young women with the skills necessary to be competent and self-assured at the postsecondary level. Planning for a college education formally begins with the transition plan, but parents should start this process as early as the seeds of high expectations for college and fulfilling careers can be planted. It is never too early to begin planning for this important step.

There are certain roadblocks to be aware of in the planning process (Lehmann, Davies, & Laurin, 2000):

- Lack of adequate disability services available at the college
- Lack of disability awareness
- Lack of sufficient financial resources
- Lack of self-advocacy skills

In order to address these roadblocks, parents, professionals, and the young woman with ASD must develop a comprehensive plan. Here are some specific guidelines to follow when preparing for postsecondary education.

1. **Plan early.** The skills required for college need to be taught throughout adolescence, so take time to teach self-determination. According to the National Council on Disabilities (2000), many students with disabilities enter postsecondary education with an inability to identify their needs and to recognize their own disability and advocate for services.

Young women with ASD need a script to follow in order to explain their strengths and needs to college professors. Assist by role-playing and asking questions about the disability. This will require several opportunities for practice prior to the beginning of the school year. It is also necessary for the student to understand the shift of power between parents and child upon entering college. No longer can the parents advocate and request accommodations. The student is ultimately responsible for requesting services and disclosing her disability.

2. **Pick the right school.** There are many options for postsecondary education – from traditional four-year schools to community colleges, public versus private schools, as well as vocational schools. Determine the right match by touring the school and meeting with advisors and faculty, preferably at various programs. Inquire about their services for students with disabilities. It is important that young women with ASD are able to articulate their disability needs and ask questions of advisors. Writing the questions down ahead of time is helpful.

By Marla Comm

From *Women from Another Planet* (2003)

The only things I found hard in my undergraduate days were exams held in the evening, which interrupted my supper routine. I always needed and still need that routine to give me something pleasurable enough at the end of the day to keep me going through the rest of the day. I used to try to get out of class by feigning illness, but that only worked twice. (p. 234)

3. **Review coursework.** As we can see from Marla's story, it is important to review the class schedule and select the best times for taking certain courses. Some young women with ASD experience sensory issues with large classes or with the lighting of the classroom. This should be taken into consideration when selecting a college. It is also important to make sure there is plenty of time between classes to address transportation needs.

Nondiscrimination in Postsecondary Institutions

Section 504 of the Vocational Rehabilitation Act of 1973 and the Americans with Disabilities Act (ADA) protect postsecondary students from discrimination. Although colleges and universities are not required by law to provide a free appropriate public education, they must provide appropriate academic adjustments as necessary to ensure that they do not discriminate on the basis of disability. Appropriate academic adjustments include reducing course loads, providing note-takers, recording devices, and extended time for test-taking. They are not required to lower the essential requirements of a course or make changes that would fundamentally alter the nature of the course.

(Office of Civil Rights: www.ed.gov/about/offices/list/ocr)

4. **Provide documentation to receive services.** Parents and professionals should keep meticulous records of high school meetings, transition plans, and IEP documents, as these documents are crucial in acquiring special services in public colleges. Although an IEP may not be the only documentation required by the university, it will assist staff in planning reasonable academic adjustments. Young women with ASD should apply for modifications to courses as early as possible. Vocational Rehabilitation centers can also be of assistance when planning for college and determining the necessary modifications. They may offer free seminars or services to individuals with disabilities who are preparing for postsecondary education.

Mon.ey [muhn-ee] Simply pronouncing the word sends chills down my spine. I always understood the concept of finance, but lacked the filter necessary to budget properly. Luckily, I enlisted my parents' help a few years ago, and their guidance was exceedingly constructive.

Other young adults took advantage of my desire to fit in by continually bumming money from me, expecting me to pay for various items, and conveniently glancing away when the dinner bill arrived. In return, I received false flattery and acceptance (until the cash flow ceased). My parents bravely volunteered their support after witnessing the depression I endured as a result of my growing financial burden. They started a checking and savings account on my behalf, sat down and discussed my budget, and laid down the rules. I had no debit card and was instead given a weekly allowance in cash. If I wanted to make a purchase outside the allotted budget, I had to consult my father. He became my voice of reason. The impulse purchases stopped. My parents provided immeasurable help for almost two years, until I married and assumed full responsibility for my own finances. My husband now shields me from those who might take advantage of me and helps me understand the discipline required to maintain a budget.

5. **Teach money and time management skills.** As illustrated in Jana's story, money and time management skills pose challenges for many young women with ASD. Therefore, it is important to repeatedly review these skills when entering a new arena. Most will need assistance creating a budget and prioritizing

schedules, for example. This may be an appropriate time to begin using an electronic organizer (PDA). This technology can help plan the day and write lists for upcoming papers and exams. PDAs also have electronic alarms that can remind a student when to go to class or when it is time to study.

By Charlotte (age 32 with ASD)

If you know that you have Asperger's and you're in high school or college, I think that it would be beneficial to find a cause in which to get involved. Don't feel discouraged because others make fun of you or if you're unpopular. Remember, you may have this disorder, but it is not who you are. There are many ways for girls with ASD to connect socially. Join the fight against cancer, homelessness, or AIDS. Tutor young children in reading.

When I was in high school, I started a magazine drive for patients at our local hospital. People would place their old magazines in a box in the school office. I would load them into my car once a week and then put them on a cart at the hospital and deliver them to patients on Saturdays. Originally, I did this kind of volunteer work to put on my college applications, but it led to being a source of great fulfillment for me.

Charlotte provides us with some additional advice for young women with ASD who might be entering college and are preparing for a positive experience. Parents, professionals, and the young woman with ASD must candidly and explicitly address self-advocacy, disclosure, and requesting academic adjustments to meet her unique needs. The team must also design a postsecondary program that includes carefully selected coursework and address the adaptive skills necessary to meet the young woman's needs for everyday living. The goal for college is future employment in an area of interest, financial independence, and personal fulfillment. With proper planning and support, this goal can become a reality for many.

The Working Girl

By Charlotte (age 32 with ASD)

When my father retired, my parents moved to Nevada. I basically came along with the luggage. I didn't have a choice; without a decent-paying job, I couldn't stay in New York. Shortly after arriving in Las Vegas, I got a job at a department store. What a let-down that was from what I had imagined for myself. I felt like I was a lab rat, with everyone saying, "Let's see what happens to her this time. Maybe she won't get fired for a change." After eight months of working at the store, my Asperger's came out again. I insulted a coworker, telling her that she "stunk" and that it was very selfish of her to come to work with an odor problem. When you have Asperger's you don't realize that what you are saying is inappropriate when you say it.

Preparing young women with ASD for employment requires more than just focusing on entry-level job skills. For example,

Jana had the basic skills for seeking competitive employment but still required the social skills for getting along on the job. Parents should work closely with the high school transition team when planning for future employment.

By Zosia Zaks

From *Life and Love* (2006)

Many of us have difficulty socializing on the job partially because social interaction requires extra energy and partially because we may not know how to interact appropriately for all the different situations that arise. Interacting with the public, for example, requires a worker to modulate his voice, his social approach, and his topics of conversation according to the customer. (p. 149)

Ms. Zaks articulates an important purpose of transition planning. The scope of the transition plan should not only address specific job skills but also the social and communication skills that are necessary for a successful employment experience.

According to the U.S. Department of Labor (www.bls.gov), employers are looking for well-rounded individuals who can get along in a variety of settings and work well with people. The top 10 critical employability skills are:

1. Communication
2. Honesty/integrity
3. Teamwork
4. Interpersonal skills

5. Motivation/initiative

6. Strong work ethic

7. Analytical skills

8. Flexibility/adaptability

9. Computer skills

10. Time management/organizational skills

Each of these skills should be assessed, and areas that need improvement should be addressed in the transition plan and be subject to further development. Employers are not only looking for basic skills to complete a job but are searching for employees who can add value to the work environment. Jana had the skills to effectively do her job at the department store, but she lacked the skills for dealing with her coworkers. In order to prevent this type of scenario, several steps can be implemented beginning early in high school.

1. **Brainstorm areas of interests.** Everyone has specific areas of interests that can lead to future employment. Make a list of all areas of interest and, with the assistance of the guidance counselor, create a list of all jobs that encompass those areas. Do not limit the possibilities, have high expectations.

   Teachers play an important role in assisting young girls in career exploration and interest inventories. This is the beginning of the job-matching process. There are many new computer programs and websites available to help young people to search out possible areas of interests and career assessments; for example, www.bls.gov/k12 and www.yesjobsearch.com

By Temple Grandin

From *Unwritten Rules of Social Relationships* (2005)

I cannot emphasize enough the importance of finding and then developing a talent area in children with ASD that can be turned into a viable profession such as drafting, commercial art, custom cabinet work, fixing cars or computer programming. These efforts provide an opportunity for a person to have an intellectually satisfying career. (p. 26)

2. **Seek out volunteer work.** Working as a volunteer is a great place to start for young women with ASD. Network with businesses or non-profit agencies that have volunteer opportunities within their specific areas of interest. Volunteer work will allow them to hone in on employability skills and work on areas that may need improvement. Volunteer work is often less stressful and allows more flexibility for learning social skills on the job. Volunteer work also is an asset when writing a resume.

3. **Identify possible job coaches and mentors.** A job coach is critically important when first seeking employment. A job coach can assist in providing a link between the employer and the employee. The job coach does more than just support the employee, and can help to educate others about the disability and the needs of the employee (Hawkins, 2004). To find a job coach, speak with the school guidance counselor, a representative of Vocational Rehabilitation, or your local autism/Asperger support group or non-profit agency.

> ### Vocational Rehabilitation (VR)
>
> VR is a state and federal agency that provides time-limited services to individuals with disabilities. Services include employment assistance, housing needs, and medical services. Individuals must apply for services based on their needs. Contacting your state VR agency is a critical first step for identifying a positive job match and a job coach (www.ed.gov/about/offices/OSERS/RSA.html).

4. **Review disclosure skills.** As discussed earlier, disclosure is a personal decision that should be carefully considered (Shore et al., 2004). When, how, and to whom a young woman with ASD discloses her disability may make or break an employment experience. Several resources cover the topic of disclosure, for example: *The 411 on Disability Disclosure: A Workbook for Youth with Disabilities* (www.ncwd-youth.info). This workbook can assist young women and their families in preparing to disclose information about their disability.

5. **Create a checklist for "Getting Along on the Job."** The checklist should provide clear directions on specific work conditions to be targeted in the work environment. Each checklist is based on the needs of the work environment. Parents, job coaches, or a trusted friend may review the checklist on a regular basis to ensure that the rules are being followed and still apply.

Getting Along on the Job Checklist	YES	NO
On time		
Personal hygiene is adequate		
Clothing is appropriate		
Smiles and says hello to coworkers		
Talks about appropriate topics		
Maintains personal space		
Stays organized		
On task		
Completes work		

By Jana (age 27 with ASD)

Working as a receptionist in a dental office is the worst job for an Aspie. I must fight insurance companies on a daily basis (automated people), rude people, rude people that don't want to pay, crazy people, frightened people, occasionally wonderful people, LOADS OF PEOPLE! Oftentimes, I hold my tongue to remain professional, but it's difficult and mentally draining. Having interacted with such a diverse cross-section of humans, I feel confident in most situations, but I would recommend a less social job for Aspies.

The Interview

Job interviews can be wrought with anxiety and mistakes. There are many great resources in books, on the Internet, and at the local library on preparing for the interview. Take it a step further and role-play the interview process. Parents and professionals can play the part of the future employer, and the young woman with ASD can practice her interview skills. For extra teaching opportunities, videotape the practice session and use the video as a teaching tool.

We can learn a lot about the importance of preparing for the world of competitive employment from Jana's story. A positive job match is crucial. Parents and professionals must investigate all aspects of the work environment, including sensory and social needs (Hurlbutt & Chalmers, 2004). As illustrated, Jana's skills did not match the requirements of the job. After brainstorming possible employment opportunities, the list should be narrowed down based on the strengths and weaknesses of the young woman with ASD and the demands of the job. Temple Grandin (2005, p. 26) has said it best "My life would not be worth living if I did not have intellectually satisfying work. My career is my life." This should be the goal for all young women with ASD.

Conclusion

Life is one long transition that we have to be prepared to embrace. In this chapter we have reviewed some of the pertinent issues for young women with ASD. Self-determination and self-advocacy skills are the foundation for lifelong success in college, the world of work, and living independently. Parents and professionals continue to play an important role in supporting young women with ASD and teaching them the skills for dating, networking within their community, and finding viable employment. The experiences and strategies discussed in this chapter, as provided from other parents and adult women with ASD, are invaluable. Being able to properly care for themselves and develop effective coping skills will enable girls with ASD to become their own advocates in preparing for a successful future.

CHAPTER 5

Oh, the Places You'll Go

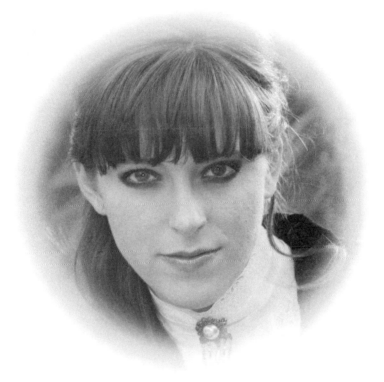

By Ashley (age 20 with ASD)

*I*t took me several years to admit that I had issues. After all the research my mom had shown me, I could definitely see that I had tendencies. But the part where I didn't see eye-to-eye with the experts is that I believe Asperger Syndrome isn't a disorder. It's a gift. Unlike the rest of the world, we can excel in mathematics, science, the arts, etc., all with half the effort *everyone else needs. That is why there are such great minds as Einstein, Bach, and Mozart. I love the fact that I can get through college with a 3.8 GPA without taking notes or staying up until 2 a.m. studying. It may take me a little longer than the average person to learn how to behave socially, but this skill can be rote taught. It can become habit. I can step back and watch the rest of the world and observe what irritates people, what reactions are the most efficient, and what people have accepted as the norm. Natural academic ability is not something at which you can work. You either have it, or you don't. Some may view Asperger's as a curse, but I wouldn't trade it for the world!!!*

Findings

The future for girls with ASD is unlimited and boundless. This chapter will provide the authors' insights based on 12 years of parenting a young girl with ASD, 22 years of working in special education, and endless hours of inspired interviews with girls with ASD and their families. We have reviewed the research, however limited, on this important topic and would like to share our findings to assist parents, professionals, and girls with ASD in navigating their journey.

After an exhaustive review of the most salient issues and practical strategies for girls with ASD, we share suggestions for creating long-term positive outcomes, which include promoting self-worth and independence, focusing on education, planning for the future, embracing uniqueness, and creating a network of support.

Maintain High Expectations

First, we must create opportunities for promoting positive self-worth and independence. Ashley's philosophy about Asperger Syndrome at the opening of this chapter should be an inspiration for other girls with ASD. Ashley states that Asperger's is not a disorder but a gift. She did not use ASD as an excuse, but built on her strengths and talents to achieve her goals. Although ASD can be challenging both academically and socially, if a girl focuses on her abilities, not disabilities, she can accomplish beyond her dreams.

As parents and professionals, we cannot let our own fears inhibit our girls' personal growth and independence. We need to accept and validate their uniqueness. All accomplishments should be valued – whether big or small. This will build their self-esteem and encourage them to try new challenges. There are many ways to guide them in discovering their talents or interests. One idea is to expose our daughters to a variety of experiences through volunteering at local organizations and active involvement in extracurricular activities. This might also help steer them down the path of future employment.

Seek Knowledge

Our second finding is the need for a focus on education for parents, professionals, and girls with ASD. Parents must first educate themselves on the disability of ASD. Parents must review the most current scientific and reliable research and seek out professional assistance on early diagnosis. Parents are their child's advocates must be acquainted with best-practice standards, the laws pertaining to their child, and the child's and family's rights to accessing appropriate services.

Professionals must also seek ongoing training and education. School professionals can assist parents in staying abreast of new treatment strategies. Classroom teachers should create learning environments that promote diversity and positive outcomes for all students. Professionals should ensure school environments are safe places for girls with ASD to learn. Professionals should also be positive role models and mentors for girls with ASD. The field of ASD is still in the infancy stages of research and standards; therefore, professionals must continually seek out new strategies and follow best-practice standards.

Girls with ASD must also educate themselves about their disability. Self-advocacy skills can be taught early in the child's development. Parents and professionals should begin the process of discussing the disability and its strengths and weaknesses and introducing books and biographies from people with ASD, such as books written by Temple Grandin, Liane Holliday Willey, Donna Williams, and Zosia Zaks.

Empowering girls with ASD with the knowledge of their disability will increase opportunities and outcomes. Without this knowledge, girls with ASD will be limited in potential employment and independence. Self-determination and self-advocacy are leading factors in successful outcomes for girls with ASD in all facets of life.

Plan for the Future

Our third finding relates to the need for planning for the future. As parents and professionals often struggle with the day-to-day challenges of working with girls with ASD, it is important to take time out to take a broader view of long-term outcomes. We are frequently forced to seek immediate answers to problem behaviors: "How do I get her to eat?" "How can I get her to do her homework?" and "How do I help her take the test?"

Although the answers to these questions are important, we must step back now and again and look beyond these immediate needs and into the future. "How do I make sure she will graduate?" "How can I help her date?" and "How can I assist her in getting a job?" These questions will assist everybody – the child, the school team, and the parents – in focusing on the future.

Planning for the future requires that all members of the team have high expectations and not limit themselves by stereotypes. Negative public perceptions of disabilities and gender stereotypes can present multiple barriers to future planning. "Only when issues of gender are addressed can we be sure that women are being accurately diagnosed and that they are receiving help and support tailored to their unique position in life and in society" (Zaks, 2006, p. 303).

Parents and professionals must actively fight against such limiting ideas. Girls with ASD can achieve great success in personal and professional relationships when we actively fight against narrow-minded ideas. With appropriate and creative planning, successful employment in their chosen field, meaningful relationships, and lifelong independence are all possible outcomes for girls with ASD.

Although all plans for the future should include elements for acquiring job skills, social skills, and personal independence, each plan is uniquely designed to meet the needs of the individual girl with ASD. Plans should be written in broad terms and with loosely assigned timeframes. Arbitrary goals and rigid timelines can lead to disappointment and, eventually, a feeling of failure. Girls with ASD will acquire specific skills and goals at different stages and should be supported throughout their development in achieving their goals. Also, as girls get older, they should become active participants in directing their future planning with the assistance of a support team.

Embrace Uniqueness

Our fourth finding suggests that we embrace the uniqueness and positive qualities of girls with ASD. The disparity between males and females in being diagnosed, receiving special education services, and long-term employment rates suggests that we must actively fight against stereotypes and narrow-minded thinking. These roadblocks can have profound effects on future outcomes. Parents and professionals can support girls with ASD by taking pride in their accomplishments and supporting their unique interests.

Part of the roles and responsibilities for parents and professionals is to accept a broader definition of what it means to be a woman with a disability, including challenging stereotypes and instilling a belief in oneself. We can also concretely teach the specific age-appropriate skills necessary for acceptance by peers in social situations and job-related social skills. Knowledge of the social rules balanced with a nurturing acceptance from others will allow girls with ASD to blossom in their own individuality.

Create a Network of Support

Lastly, we believe in the importance of creating a network of support for families and girls with ASD. Parents and professionals cannot be all things to our children. That is why it is important to enlist the help of friends, family, local community agencies, and professional organizations. Support groups are extremely beneficial for parents and professionals as a forum for sharing their stories and knowledge with other families. Networking with people of similar circumstances often brings relief that you are not alone in your journey. Each person's experience can have a positive impact on other support group members by validating their feelings and providing them with understanding and acceptance.

Our girls with ASD also need to be able to connect with their peers for support and understanding. There are many avenues for obtaining this type of service, such as Asperger-related Internet sites and local age-appropriate support groups and/or social skills groups. To become self-aware, accept their strengths and weaknesses, and form meaningful relationships, girls with ASD need to become involved with others who share the same experiences and feelings.

These findings are a summary of our thoughts and recommendations based on the current literature, interviews, and our personal and professional experience. We have organized our findings to include promoting self-worth and independence, focusing on education, planning for the future, embracing individuality and uniqueness, and creating a network of support. Although the individual needs of girls with ASD will dictate the level of support and the priority of each finding, we hope to have provided a framework for achieving long-term success and positive outcomes.

Conclusion

Traditionally, researchers have looked at disability-specific characteristics with a disregard for gender. Girls with ASD tend to be more withdrawn and anxious than boys and may not be seen as needing educational services. Without adequate diagnosis and services, girls and young women with ASD will blame themselves for their inabilities. They will endure silently.

> I am convinced that girls on the spectrum fly under the radar far too easily, getting by until survival techniques no longer work. Most little girls try hard not to interrupt, they want to look pretty and well groomed, they tend to stay in their seats, they tend to withdraw instead of making a scene. As adults, autistic women may seem weird, lost in their own worlds, unusually withdrawn or alone, rebellious or wallowing in self-pity, while the true struggle – dealing with the challenges of autism – goes unrecognized. Again, I'm not a scientist, but even if more males than females are autistic, I think many women are missing from the count and losing out on valuable chances to learn skill sets that can be the difference between healthy self-esteem and confidence or trouble and danger. (Zaks, 2006, p. 303)

In general, girls are not receiving the services they need to benefit from instruction and live independent and self-fulfilling lives. Girls are failing to be noticed due to gender stereotypes (Hoffschmidt & Weinstein, 2003). Girls are underrepresented in the ASD community. It appears from the research that they must demonstrate significant levels of disability before their needs are recognized. In writing this book, we hope to have changed this way of thinking. We want to create an urgency in the autism community for all parents and professionals to seek a change in diagnosing and providing services for girls with ASD.

One day they may find a more scientific and accurate way to look at how people's brains work to establish what sort of difficulties they may have, and when that day comes, maybe it will result in more females getting diagnosed. In the meantime, only increased awareness of females on the autistic spectrum will help us not to be simply disregarded as freakish anomalies and not abundant enough to be worthy of consideration. We do exist.

– Anonymous

A Little Secret

By Amanda (age 11 with ASD)

She looks like any other little girl.
But she holds a secret you might never suspect.
There is something different about her.
She often talks about Ancient Egypt and nothing else, even if you
don't want to hear about it.
She is very well meaning, but frequently misunderstood.
Some say she is a "little professor."
She knows a lot about what interests her.
Her clothes bother her a lot.
Just a little tag might feel like sand paper.
Food needs to taste and smell just right or she won't eat it.
She thinks she can't go a week without ice cream.
Noise in the lunchroom really gets to be confusing, and
She wants to say BE QUIET!!!!!
Light......... is 100 times brighter to her.
Oh, what a world she lives in.

What is this little secret she holds?

It's called Asperger's Syndrome, a high-functioning form of autism.
Many people are suspected of having it: Einstein, Michael Angelo.
1 out every 166 children will be diagnosed with autism this year.

How do I know so much about Asperger's Syndrome?
I know because I have it.
Some say it is a disability.
But I am a girl with dreams.
I will take what God has given me
Along with the challenge and use it
To fulfill the purpose He has for me.
Let me say to you,
If you know someone who seems a little different
Look for something good.
It will be there.
It may be just "a little secret" waiting to be told.
A dream waiting to unfold.

References

American Association of University Women. (2004). *Women and girls with disabilities.* Washington, DC: AAUW Educational Foundation and National Education Association.

Attwood, T. (1999). *The pattern of abilities and development of girls with Asperger's Syndrome.* www.tonyattwood.com

Attwood, T. (2007). *The complete guide to Asperger's Syndrome.* London: Jessica Kingsley Publishers.

Ayers, A. J. (1989). *Sensory integration and praxis test.* Los Angeles: Western Psychological Services.

Baker, J. (2003). *Social skills training for children and adolescents with Asperger Syndrome and social-communication problems.* Shawnee Mission, KS: Autism Asperger Publishing Company.

Baron-Cohen, S. (1995). *Mindblindness.* London: The MIT Press.

Bashe, P. R., & Kirby, B. (2001). *The oasis guide to Asperger Syndrome: Advice, support, insights, and inspiration.* New York: Crown Publishers.

Bellini, S. (2006). *Building social relationships – A systematic approach to teaching social interaction skills to children and adolescents with autism spectrum disorders and other social difficulties.* Shawnee Mission, KS: Autism Asperger Publishing Company.

Besag, V. (2006). Bullying among girls: Friend or foes. *School Psychology International, 27*(5), 535-551.

Biel, L. (2005). Sensory issues and the IEP. *Autism Asperger's Digest,* September/October, 10-11.

Cardon, T. (2004). *Let's talk emotions. Helping children with social cognitive deficits, including AS, HFA, and NVLD, learn to understand and express empathy and emotions.* Shawnee Mission, KS: Autism Asperger Publishing Company.

Coloroso, B. (2003). *The bully, the bullied, and the bystander.* New York: Harper Resource.

Coucouvanis, J. (2005*). Super skills: A social skills group program for children with Asperger Syndrome, high-functioning autism and related challenges.* Shawnee Mission, KS: Autism Asperger Publishing Company.

Crompton, V., & Kessner, E. (2003). *Saving beauty from the beast.* Boston: Little, Brown and Company.

Crowder, C. (2002). *Eating, sleeping, and getting up.* New York: Broadway Books.

Cutler, E. (2004). *A thorn in my pocket.* Arlington, TX: Future Horizons.

Debbault, D. (2003). *Safety issues for adolescents with Asperger Syndrome.* In L. Holliday Willey (Ed.), *Asperger syndrome in adolescence* (pp. 148-178). London: Jessica Kingsley Publishers.

Dunn, M. A. (2006). *S.O.S. – Social skills in our schools: A social skills program for children with pervasive developmental disorders, including high-functioning autism and Asperger Syndrome, and their typical peers.* Shawnee Mission, KS: Autism Asperger Publishing Company.

Dunn, W. (1999). *The sensory profile.* San Antonio, TX: The Psychological Corporation.

Ebeling, D., Deschenes, C., & Sprague, J. (1994). *Adapting curriculum and instruction in inclusive classrooms.* Bloomington, IN: Institute for the Study of Developmental Disabilities.

Ernsperger, L. (2003). *Keys to success for teaching students with autism.* Arlington, TX: Future Horizons.

Ernsperger, L., & Stegen-Hanson, T. (2004). *Just take a bite: Easy, effective answers to food aversions and eating challenges.* Arlington, TX: Future Horizons.

Feiges, L. S., & Weiss, M. J. (2004). *Sibling stories – Reflections on life with a brother or sister on the autism spectrum.* Shawnee Mission, KS: Autism Asperger Publishing Company.

Fine, M., & Asch, A. (1988). *Women with disabilities.* Philadelphia: Temple University Press.

Frith, U. (Ed.). (1991). *Autism and Asperger Syndrome.* London: Jessica Kingsley Publishers.

Frohoff, K. (2004). A team approach to transitioning students with autism from elementary school to middle school. *Autism Asperger's Digest,* July/August, 16-21.

Gillberg, C. (1991). *Clinical and neurobiological aspects of Asperger Syndrome in six family studies.* In U. Frith (Ed.), *Autism and Asperger syndrome* (pp. 123-146). Cambridge, UK: Cambridge University Press.

Grandin, T., & Barron, S. (2005). *The unwritten rules of social relationships.* Arlington, TX: Future Horizons.

Grandin, T., & Duffy, K. (2004). *Developing talents: Careers for individuals with Asperger Syndrome and high-functioning autism.* Shawnee Mission, KS: Autism Asperger Publishing Company.

Gray, C. (1995). *Social Stories™ unlimited: Social stories and comic strip conversations.* Jenison, MI: Jenison Public Schools.

Gray, C. (2004). Gray's guide to bullying. *Jenison Autism Journal, 16*(1), 1-59.

Gurian, M. (2002). *The wonder of girls: Understanding the hidden nature of our daughters.* New York: Atria Books.

Hall, M., Kleinert, H., & Kearns, J. (2000). Going to college: Postsecondary programs for students with moderate and severe disabilities. *Teaching Exceptional Children, 32*(3), 58-65.

Harris, S., & Glasberg, B. (2003). *Siblings of children with autism: A guide for families.* Bethesda, MD: Woodbine House.

Hart, S. (2001). *Preventing sibling rivalry.* New York: The Free Press.

Hawkins, G. (2004). *How to find work that works for people with Asperger Syndrome.* London: Jessica Kingsley Publishers.

Heinrichs, R. (2003). *Perfect targets: Asperger Syndrome and bullying – Practical solutions for surviving the social world.* Shawnee Mission, KS: Autism Asperger Publishing Company.

Hoffman, C., Sweeney, D., Gilliam, J., & Lopez-Wagner, M. (2006). Sleep problems in children with autism and typically developing children. *Focus on Autism and Other Developmental Disabilities, 21*(3), 146-152.

Hoffschmidt, S., & Weinstein, C. (2003). Women with visible and invisible disabilities. *Women and Therapy, 26*(2), 81-91.

Hurlbutt, K., & Chalmers, L. (2004). Employment and adults with Asperger Syndrome. *Focus on Autism and Other Developmental Disabilities, 19*(4), 215-222.

Kanner, L. (1943). Autistic disturbances of affective contact. *Nervous Child, 2,* 217-250.

Kopp, S., & Gillberg, C. (1992). Girls with social deficits and learning problems: Autism, atypical Asperger Syndrome or a variant of these conditions. *European Child and Adolescent Psychiatry, 1*(2), 89-99.

Kranowitz, C. (1998). *The out-of-sync child*. New York: The Berkley Publishing Group.

Krueger, A. (2001). *Guide to toilet training*. New York: Ballantine Books.

Lehmann, J., Davies, T., & Laurin, K. (2000). Listening to student voices about postsecondary education. *Teaching Exceptional Children, 32*(5), 60-65.

Lonsdale, S. (1997). *Women and disability*. New York: St. Martin Press.

Lord, C., Schopler, E., & Revicki, D. (1982). Sex differences in autism. *Journal of Autism and Developmental Disorders, 12*(4), 317-329.

Lynch, R., & Gussel, L. (1996). Disclosure and self-advocacy regarding disability-related needs: Strategies to maximize integration in postsecondary education. *Journal of Counseling and Development, 74*(4), 352-364.

Marks, S., Schrader, C., Levine, M., Hagie, C., Longaker, T., Morales, M., & Peters, I. (1999). Social skills for social ills. *Teaching Exceptional Children, 32*(2), 56-61.

Martin, R. (2003). Pace V. Bogalusa city school board: Implications for parents. *Autism Asperger's Digest,* July/August, 44-47.

Mayes, S. D., & Calhoun, S. L. (1999). Symptoms of autism in young children and correspondence with the DSM. *Infants and Young Children, 12*(1), 90-97.

McAfee, J. (2002). *Navigating the social world*. Arlington, TX: Future Horizons.

McHugh, M. (1999). *Special siblings: Growing up with someone with a disability*. New York: Hyperion.

McNamara, B., & McNamara, F. (1997). *Keys to dealing with bullies*. Hauppauge, NY: Barron's Educational Services.

Meyer, D. (2004). What siblings want parents and service providers to know. *Advocate, 37*(4), 24-26.

Miller, J. K. (2003). *Women from another planet: Our lives in the universe of autism*. Bloomington, IN: A Dancing Mind Book.

Mishna, F. (2003). Learning disabilities and bullying: Double jeopardy. *Journal of Learning Disabilities, 36*(4), 336-347.

Murkoff, H., Eisenberg, A., & Hathaway, S. (2003). *What to expect the first year*. New York: Workman Publishing.

Myles, B. S., & Adreon, D. (2001). *Asperger Syndrome and adolescence: Practical solutions for school success*. Shawnee Mission, KS: Autism Asperger Publishing Company.

Myles, B. S., & Southwick, J. (2005). *Asperger Syndrome and difficult moments: Practical strategies for tantrums, rage, and meltdowns*. Shawnee Mission, KS: Autism Asperger Publishing Company.

Myles, B. S., Trautman, M., & Schelvan, R. (2004). *The hidden curriculum*. Shawnee Mission, KS: Autism Asperger Publishing Company.

National Center for Injury Prevention and Control. www.cdc.gov/ncipc

National Council on Disabilities. www.ncd.gov

National Research Council. (2001). *Educating children with autism*. Washington, DC: National Academy Press.

Nyden, A., Hjelmquist, E., & Gillberg, C. (2000). Autism spectrum and attention disorders in girls. *European Child & Adolescent Psychiatry, 9*(1), 180-185.

Pantley, E. (2005). *The no cry sleep solution*. New York: McGraw Hill.

Pantley, E. (2007). *The no cry potty training solution.* New York: McGraw Hill.

Reisman, J., & Hanschu, B. (1992). *Sensory integration inventory.* Hugo, MN: PDP Press.

Resources for Rehabilitation. (1994). *A women's guide to coping with disability.* Lexington, MA: Author.

Richard, G. (1997). *The source for autism.* East Moline, IL: Linguisystems.

Rousso, H., & Wehmeyer, M. (2001). *Double jeopardy: Addressing gender equity in special education.* New York: State University of New York Press.

Rousso, H., & Wehmeyer, M. (2002). *Gender matters: Training for educators working with students with disabilities.* Newton, MA: Education Development Center.

Sakai, K. (2005). *Finding our way: Practical solutions for creating a supportive home and community for the Asperger Syndrome family.* Shawnee Mission, KS: Autism Asperger Publishing Company.

Shaw, V. (1999). *A girl's guide to what's happening to your body.* New York: Rosen Publishing Group.

Shield, J., & Mullen, M. (2002). *Healthy eating for kids.* Hoboken, NJ: John Wiley & Sons.

Shore, S. (Ed.). (2004). *Ask and tell: Self-advocacy and disclosure for people on the autism spectrum.* Shawnee Mission, KS: Autism Asperger Publishing Company.

Smith, T. (1997). Sexual differences in pervasive developmental disorders. *Medscape Psychiatry and Mental Health e-Journal, 2*(3).

Sugai, G., & Lewis, T. (1996). Preferred and promising practices for social skills instruction. *Focus on Exceptional Children, 29*(4), 1-16.

Summers, L. (2006). *Autism in not a life sentence: How one family took on autism and won.* Shawnee Mission, KS: Autism Asperger Publishing Company.

Test, D., Karvonen, M., Wood, W., Browder, D., & Algozzine, B. (2000). Choosing a self-determination curriculum. *Teaching Exceptional Children, 33*(2), 48-53.

Twachtman-Cullen, D. (2002). Bullying in the classroom. *Advocate, 35*(4), 29-31.

Voors, W. (2000). *The parent's book about bullying.* Center City, MN: Hazelden.

Wagner, S. (2002). *Inclusive programming for middle school students with autism/Asperger's Syndrome.* Arlington, TX: Future Horizons.

Walker, H., Colvin, G., & Ramsey, E. (1995). *Antisocial behavior in school: School strategies and best practice.* Pacific Grove, CA: Brooks/Cole Publishing Company.

Wehmeyer, M., & Schwartz, M. (1997). Self-determination and positive adult outcomes. *Exceptional Children, 63*, 245-255.

Weissbluth, M. (1999). *Healthy sleep habits, happy child.* New York: Ballantine Publishing Group.

Willey, L. H. (1999). *Pretending to be normal: Living with Asperger's Syndrome.* London: Jessica Kingsley Publishers.

Wing, L. (2001). *The autistic spectrum: A parent's guide to understanding and helping your child.* Berkeley, CA: Ulysses Press.

Wolraich, M. (2003). *Guide to toilet training.* New York: Bantam Books.

Zaks, Z. (2006). *Life and love: Positive strategies for autistic adults.* Shawnee Mission, KS: Autism Asperger Publishing Company.

Appendix

Additional Resources and Websites

The following is a list of websites and references that we have found to be useful for parents and professionals. The list is not exhaustive but is meant as a starting point for seeking more information.

Abilitations: www.abilitations.com

The Abilitation's catalogue provides innovative and sensory products to help educators and parents work with students of all ages. Their products provide a wide range of activities and products to help children with learning, behavioral, speech, and sensory differences achieve their full potential.

American Girl Series of Books: www.americangirls.com

American Girl's mission is to celebrate girls by embracing who they are today and looking forward to who they will become tomorrow. Through an array of premium-quality books, dolls, clothes, toys, and accessories, American Girl has earned the loyalty of millions of girls and the praise and trust of parents and educators. American Girl books are there for girls every step of the way – as they begin to read, start school, face issues about friends and family, and dream about setting off on their own adventures. The American Girl's books provide a "head-to-toe" guide that answers all a girl's questions about her changing body, from hair care to healthy eating, bad breath to bras, periods to pimples, and everything in between.

American Occupational Therapy Association: www.aota.org
The American Occupational Therapy Association (AOTA) is the nationally recognized professional association of more than 35,000 occupational therapists, occupational therapy assistants, and students of occupational therapy. Practitioners work with people experiencing health problems such as stroke, spinal cord injuries, cancer, congenital conditions, developmental problems, and mental illness. Occupational therapy helps people regain, develop, and build skills that are essential for independent functioning, health, and well-being.

American Speech-Language-Hearing Association: www.asha.org
The American Speech-Language-Hearing Association (ASHA) is the professional, scientific, and credentialing association for more than 127,000 members and affiliates who are speech-language pathologists, audiologists, and speech, language, and hearing scientists in the United States and internationally. The mission of the American Speech-Language-Hearing Association is to promote the interests of and provide the highest quality services for professionals in audiology, speech-language pathology, and speech and hearing science, and to advocate for people with communication disabilities.

Autism Society of America: www.autism-society.org
The Autism Society of America (ASA) is dedicated to increasing public awareness about autism and the day-to-day issues faced by

individuals with autism, their families, and the professionals with whom they interact. ASA and its local chapters share a common mission of providing information and education, supporting research, and advocating for programs and services for the autism community. ASA is the oldest and largest grassroots organization within the autism community. Today, more than 120,000 members and supporters are connected through a working network of nearly 200 chapters nationwide. ASA membership continues to grow as more and more parents and professionals unite to form a collective voice representing the autism community.

Bellini, S. (2006). *Building Social Relationships.* **Shawnee Mission, KS: Autism Asperger Publishing Company.**
This book addresses the need for social programming for children and adolescents with ASD by providing a comprehensive five-step model. The model incorporates the following five steps: assess social functioning, distinguish between skill acquisition and performance deficits, select intervention strategies, implement intervention, and evaluate and monitor progress.

Cardon, T. (2004). *Let's Talk Emotions: Helping Children with Social Cognitive Deficits, Including AS, HFA, and NVLD, Learn to Understand and Express Empathy and Emotions.* **Shawnee Mission, KS: Autism Asperger Publishing Company.**
The purpose of this book is to guide and help parents, teachers, and others teach their children with social cognition deficits. Through the activities included in the book, children learn to identify and respond to their own feelings as well as the feelings of others.

Durand, M. (1997). *Sleep Better: A Guide to Improving Sleep for Children with Special Needs*. Baltimore: Brookes Publishing Company.

This book offers professionals and parents, in a step-by-step approach, "how-to" instructions for addressing a variety of sleep-related problems. These widely tested, largely drug-free techniques have helped hundreds of children with special needs.

Shore S. (Ed.). (2004). *Ask and Tell: Self-Advocacy and Disclosure for People on the Autism Spectrum*. Shawnee Mission, KS: Autism Asperger Publishing Company.

This book aims to help people with autism effectively self-advocate in their pursuit of independent, productive, and fulfilling lives. The book speaks to the issue of self-advocacy and disclosure for people with autism.

Heinrichs, R. (2003). *Perfect Targets: Asperger Syndrome and Bullying*. Shawnee Mission, KS: Autism Asperger Publishing Company.

This book takes an honest look at the different types of bullying and the actions adults must take to curb bullying, helping prevent the often lifelong effects of this insidious form of behavior on victims.

Lili Claire Foundation: www.liliclairefoundation.org
The Lili Claire Foundation is a national organization established to enhance the lives of children living with neurogenetic conditions affecting their physical, intellectual, and behavioral development such as Williams Syndrome, Down Syndrome, fetal alcohol syndrome, and autism, while providing hope and resources for the families that love them.

Las Vegas Lili Claire Family Resource Center
522 E Twain Avenue
Las Vegas, NV 89169
(702)862-8141
jbradley@liliclairefoundation.org

UCLA Lili Claire Family Resource Center
300 Medical Building Plaza, Suite 1200
Los Angeles, CA 90095
(310)794-9516
staff@liliclairefoundation.org

Vanderbilt Kennedy Family Outreach Center
1810 Edgehill Avenue
Nashville, TN 37212
(615)936-5118
familyoutreach@vanderbilt.edu

National Information Center for Children and Youth with Disabilities: www.nichcy.org
NICHCY is the National Dissemination Center for Children with Disabilities. It serves the United States, Puerto Rico, and the U.S. territories, providing families, students, educators, and others with information on topics regarding children and youth with disabilities, birth through 22. This includes research-based information about effective practices for educating and providing services to children with disabilities, information about how the No Child Left Behind Act (NCLB) affects children with disabilities, and information about educational research programs and initiatives involving children with disabilities.

Office of Special Education Programs: www.ed.gov/about/offices/list/osers/osep

The Office of Special Education Programs (OSEP) is dedicated to improving results for infants, toddlers, children, and youth with disabilities ages birth through 21 by providing leadership and financial support to assist states and local districts. OSEP administers the Individuals with Disabilities Education Act (IDEA). IDEA authorizes formula grants to states and discretionary grants to institutions of higher education and other nonprofit organizations to support research, demonstrations, technical assistance and dissemination, technology and personnel development, and parent-training and information centers.

Sibling Support Project: www.siblingsupport.org

The Sibling Support Project is a national effort dedicated to the life-long concerns of brothers and sisters of people who have special health, developmental, or mental health concerns. The Sibling Support Project is the only national effort dedicated to the interests of over six million brothers and sisters of people with special health, mental health, and developmental needs.

Stop Bullying: www.bullying.org

This website is dedicated to increase the awareness of, and the problems associated with, bullying and to preventing, resolving, and eliminating bullying.

Timetimer: www.timetimer.com

A visual tool to illustrate elapsed time, the Time Timer encourages efficient use of time and provides visual ownership of time.

Willey, Liane Holliday: www.aspie.com

All of her life, Liane Holliday Willey knew she was different, but only after one of her family members was diagnosed with Asperger Syndrome, a very high-functioning form of autism, did Liane realize the reason behind her differences; she too was diagnosed with Asperger Syndrome. With the odds firmly stacked against her, Liane rose to the challenge of life as it comes to you through the broken glass of autism, to a place where she is happy, healthy and well balanced. Today, Liane is a successful writer, editor, consultant, motivational speaker, freelance author, mother, and wife.

Wheeler, M. (1998). *Toilet Training for Individuals with Autism and Related Disorders*. Arlington, TX: Future Horizons.

Individuals with autism have been reported to be the most difficult to toilet train. This comprehensive guide for parents and teachers includes over 200 toilet-training tips supported by over 60 case examples with solutions.

Wrobel, M. (2003). *Taking Care of Myself*. Arlington, TX: Future Horizons.

This book offers curriculum that guides the child and caregiver on issues of health, hygiene, and the challenge of puberty. The curriculum is designed to address the health and safety of students with autism spectrum disorders.

Behavior Intervention Plan

Proactive Plan

A	B	C
• Antecedent • Context • Environment • Before the behavior occurs • Review what may be causing the problem behavior	• Behavior • Observable • Measurable • Specific • Target behavior • Clearly define problem behavior to be addressed	• Consequence • After the behavior occurs • Function to the student • Consider why the child is exhibiting the problem behavior

Hypothesis Statement:

(When this occurs …/The child does …/In order to …)

_____

_____

_____

Select three possible changes to the environment:

1.

2.

3.

Select three highly desirable reinforcers:

1.

2.

3.

Replacement and/or Alternative Skills

Identify one social skill, one stress-reduction skill, and/or one communication skill. Also select methods for teaching the new skill.

1. _____

2. _____

3. _____

Reactive Program

In the event the target (inappropriate behavior) occurs, describe the specific reactive strategies to be implemented:

1. _____

2. _____

3. _____

Environmental Checklist

The following inventory is an informal checklist to assist parents and professionals in creating a positive environment. Each item should be reviewed and determined appropriate in meeting the needs of the child. Not all guidelines will apply to each home setting or classroom.

	YES	NO	Action Plan
Visual and physical boundaries are defined			
Areas are labeled with picture and word			
Environment is free of clutter			
Space is provided for 1:1 teaching			
Homework area is structured			
Homework is divided into small parts			
Furniture is appropriate size			
Furniture placement defines boundaries			
Open spaces are minimized			
Sensory needs are assessed			
Materials are age-appropriate			
Quiet space is provided for break area			
Rules are posted with visual supports			
Outside distractions are minimized			
Appropriate behaviors are reinforced			
Appropriate sensory activities are available			
Carpets are used to filter noise			
Auditory cue is utilized for transitions			
Schedule is posted and visible			
Reinforcement schedules are established and utilized			
Schedule includes break time (after school)			
Schedule reflects any upcoming changes			
Transition time is included			
Schedule is well rounded with a variety of activities			

Social Skills Objectives

- Maintaining appropriate physical distance
- Accepting criticism and remaining calm
- Showing empathy
- Waiting in line
- Greeting teachers
- Asking for assistance
- Keeping hands to self
- Starting conversations
- Respecting friends
- Making an apology
- Using a normal voice
- Respecting adults
- Changing the subject of a conversation
- Joining a group
- Dealing with conflicts
- Establishing eye contact
- Following instructions from peers
- Sharing a toy
- Initiating social questions
- Offering assistance to peers
- Playing game with peer
- Staying calm when losing a game
- Introducing self to a peer
- Ending play time appropriately
- Complimenting others
- Demonstrating appropriate physical distance to a speaker
- Answering the telephone

Index

Resources and Services Provided by
Dr. Lori Ernsperger

Dr. Lori Ernsperger has over 22 years of experience working in the public schools as a school administrator, teacher, and consultant. She is an autism consultant and provides intensive training to school personnel and parents. Dr. Ernsperger also presents at a variety of national and state conferences. Topics include:

1. Identifying and Designing an Appropriate Curriculum for Students with Autism Spectrum Disorders: Solutions for Designing an Effective Classroom Environment and Selecting Curriculum
2. Implementing Effective Instructional Strategies and Reinforcement Techniques: A Focus on ABA and Discrete Trial Instruction in the Classroom
3. Proactive Strategies for Managing Problem Behaviors and Effective Answers to Data Collection in the Classroom
4. Practical Strategies for Working with Students with Asperger Syndrome and High-Functioning Autism
5. How to Get your Kids to Eat a Balanced Diet: Strategies for Addressing Food Aversions and Eating Challenges

Dr. Ernsperger's Books

1. *Keys to Success for Teaching Students with Autism* (Future Horizons, 2003). Provides practical strategies for teaching students with autism in the areas of curriculum, instruction, behavior management, and data collection.

2. *Just Take a Bite* (Future Horizons, 2004). Easy and effective answers to food aversions and eating challenges.

3. *Girls Under the Umbrella of Autism Spectrum Disorders* (AAPC, 2007).

Contact Dr. Ernsperger for your training and workshop needs:
702-616-8717 or drlori@cox.net

AΛPC

Autism Asperger Publishing Co.
P.O. Box 23173
Shawnee Mission, Kansas 66283-0173
www.asperger.net